Coronary Reperfusion
Therapy in
Clinical Practice

Coronary Reperfusion Therapy in Clinical Practice

Edited by

Freek W A Verheugt MD FESC FACC

Professor of Cardiology
Heartcenter, Department of Cardiology
University Medical Center St Radboud
Nijmegen, The Netherlands

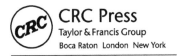

CRC Press
Taylor & Francis Group
Boca Raton London New York

CRC Press is an imprint of the
Taylor & Francis Group, an **informa** business

CRC Press
Taylor & Francis Group
6000 Broken Sound Parkway NW, Suite 300
Boca Raton, FL 33487-2742

First issued in paperback 2019

© 2006 by Taylor & Francis Group, LLC
CRC Press is an imprint of Taylor & Francis Group, an Informa business

No claim to original U.S. Government works

ISBN-13: 978-1-84184-558-6 (hbk)
ISBN-13: 978-0-367-39121-8 (pbk)

A CIP record for this book is available from the British Library.

**Visit the Taylor & Francis Web site at
http://www.taylorandfrancis.com**

**and the CRC Press Web site at
http://www.crcpress.com**

Contents

Principal contributors

Diego Ardissino
Division of Cardiology
Heart Department
Maggiore Hospital
University of Parma
Via Gramsci 14
43100 Parma
Italy

Eric Boersma
Erasmus MC Rotterdam
Department of Cardiology
Thoraxcenter
Room Ba-563
3000 CA Rotterdam
The Netherlands

Sanjaya Khanal MD FACC
Henry Ford Heart and Vascular
    Institute
Henry Ford Health System
Detroit, MI 48202
USA

Peter Klootwijk MD PhD
Erasmus MC Rotterdam
Department of Cardiology
Thoraxcenter
Room Ba-577
3000 CA Rotterdam
The Netherlands

H Roger Lijnen PhD
Center for Molecular and Vascular
    Biology
Campus Gasthuisberg, O & N
University of Leuven
Herestraat 49,
B-3000 Leuven
Belgium

Carlo Di Mario
Department of Cardiology
Royal Brompton Hospital
Sydney Street
London, SW3 6NP
UK

Freek W A Verheugt MD FESC FACC
670 Department of Cardiology
University Medical Center
10 Geert Grooteplein Center
6525 GA Nijmegen
The Netherlands

W Douglas Weaver MD FACC
Henry Ford Heart and Vascular
    Institute
Henry Ford Health System
Detroit, MI 48202
USA

Robert G Wilcox
Cardiovascular Medicine
University Hospital Nottingham
Nottingham NG7 2UH
UK

Felix Zijlstra
Department of Cardiology
Thoraxcenter
University Medical Center Groningen
Hanzeplein 1
Postbus 30.001
9700 RB Groningen
The Netherlands

Preface

Reperfusion therapy of acute myocardial infarction has been the greatest break-through in the treatment of the most important cause of death in the Western world. Better angiographic knowledge of the pathogenesis of ST segment elevation acute coronary syndrome has identified acute thrombotic occlusion of a major epicardial coronary artery as the main mechanism. This may result in catastrophic consequences such as sudden death or massive myocardial infarction.

Early reperfusion of occluded coronary arteries has been shown to improve symptoms, to enhance myocardial recovery and to improve quantity and quality of life.

There has been a dramatic evolution in reperfusion strategies: improved designs of fibrinolytic drugs and the introduction of primary coronary angioplasty. Furthermore, adjuvant therapy has been introduced and tested in numerous clinical trials. Proper patient selection, evidence-based use of fibrinolytics, balloon angioplasty, stents and adjunctive therapies form the mainstay of modern reperfusion therapies.

Coronary Reperfusion Therapy in Clinical Practice provides practical guidelines in the clinical application of fibrinolytic therapy, primary coronary angioplasty and their combination in ST segment elevation acute coronary syndrome. It is not an encyclopedia of all trials, but shows the current guidelines for physicians taking care of these acutely ill patients, whether in intensive care units, coronary care units, ambulances or emergency departments.

Freek W A Verheugt MD FESC FACC
Professor of Cardiology
Nijmegen, October 2005

1

Pharmacology of fibrinolytic agents

H Roger Lijnen and Désiré Collen

INTRODUCTION

Thrombolysis consists of the pharmacological dissolution of a blood clot by intravenous infusion of plasminogen activators that activate the fibrinolytic system. The fibrinolytic system includes a proenzyme, plasminogen, which is converted by plasminogen activators to the active enzyme plasmin, which in turn digests fibrin to soluble degradation products. Inhibition of the fibrinolytic system occurs by plasminogen activator inhibitors (mainly plasminogen activator inhibitor-1, PAI-1) and by plasmin inhibitors (mainly α_2-antiplasmin) (Figure 1.1). Thrombolytic agents that are either approved or under clinical investigation in patients with acute myocardial infarction (AMI) include streptokinase, recombinant tissue-type plasminogen activator (rt-PA or alteplase), rt-PA derivatives such as reteplase, lanoteplase and tenecteplase, anisoylated plasminogen–streptokinase activator complex (APSAC or anistreplase), two-chain urokinase-type plasminogen activator (tcu-PA or urokinase), recombinant single-chain u-PA (scu-PA or pro-urokinase, saruplase) and recombinant staphylokinase and derivatives. Fibrin-selective agents (rt-PA and derivatives, staphylokinase and derivatives and to a lesser extent scu-PA) which digest a blood clot in the absence of systemic plasminogen activation are distinguished from non-fibrin-selective agents (streptokinase, tcu-PA and APSAC) which activate systemic and fibrin-bound plasminogen relatively indiscriminately (Figure 1.1).[1] In this contribution, we review the physicochemical properties, mechanism of action and pharmacodynamics of currently available thrombolytic agents.

PHYSICOCHEMICAL PROPERTIES OF FIBRINOLYTIC AGENTS

t-PA and variants

Wild-type recombinant t-PA (rt-PA, alteplase) is obtained by expression in Chinese hamster ovary cells. It is a single-chain serine proteinase of 70 kDa, consisting of 527 amino acid residues with Ser as the NH_2-terminal amino acid; it was subsequently

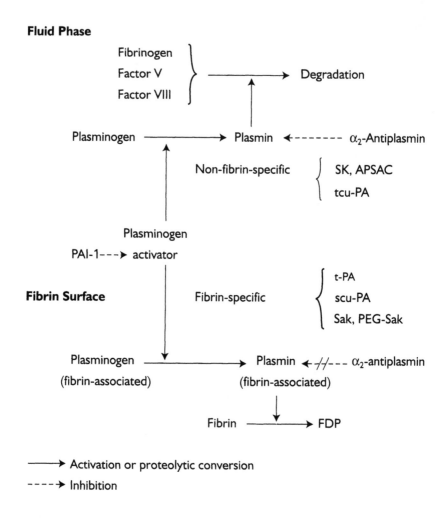

Figure 1.1 In the fibrinolytic system, the proenzyme plasminogen is activated to the active enzyme plasmin by a plasminogen activator. Plasmin degrades fibrin into soluble fibrin degradation products (FDP). Inhibition may occur at the level of the plasminogen activator (inhibition of t-PA and u-PA by plasminogen activator inhibitor-1, PAI-1), or at the level of plasmin, mainly by α_2-antiplasmin.

Non-fibrin-specific plasminogen activators (streptokinase, SK; anisoylated plasminogen streptokinase activator complex, APSAC; two-chain urokinase, tcu-PA) activate both plasminogen in the fluid phase and fibrin-associated plasminogen. Plasmin generated in the circulating blood is rapidly neutralized by α_2-antiplasmin, and excess plasmin may degrade other plasma proteins. Fibrin-specific plasminogen activators (tissue-type plasminogen activator, t-PA; single-chain u-PA, scu-PA; staphylokinase, Sak; pegylated Sak, PEG-Sak) preferentially activate fibrin-associated plasminogen. Fibrin-associated plasmin is protected from rapid inhibition by α_2-antiplasmin.

shown that native t-PA contains an NH_2-terminal extension of three amino acids, but in general the initial numbering system has been maintained. Limited plasmic hydrolysis of the Arg^{275}–Ile^{276} peptide bond converts t-PA to a two-chain molecule held together by one interchain disulfide bond. The t-PA molecule contains four domains: (1) an NH_2-terminal region of 47 residues (residues 4–50) which is homologous with the finger domains mediating the fibrin affinity of fibronectin; (2) residues 50–87 which are homologous with epidermal growth factor; (3) two kringle regions comprising residues 87–176 and 176–262 which are homologous with the five kringles of plasminogen; and (4) a serine proteinase domain (residues 276–527) with the active site residues His^{322}, Asp^{371} and Ser^{478} (Figure 1.2). The t-PA molecule comprises three potential N-glycosylation sites, at Asn^{117}, Asn^{184} and Asn^{448}.[2] In contrast to the single-chain precursor form of most serine proteinases, single-chain t-PA is enzymatically active.

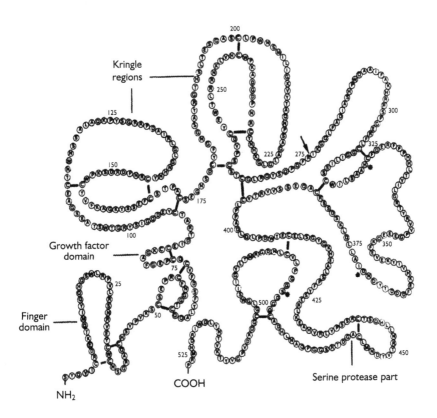

Figure 1.2 Schematic representation of the primary structure of t-PA. The amino acids are represented by their single letter symbols and black bars indicate disulfide bonds. The catalytic triad His^{322}, Asp^{371} and Ser^{478} is indicated with an asterisk. The arrow indicates the plasmin cleavage site for conversion of single-chain to two-chain t-PA.

By deletion or substitution of functional domains, by site-specific point mutations and/or by altering the carbohydrate composition, mutants of rt-PA have been produced with higher fibrin-specificity, more zymogenicity, slower clearance from the circulation and resistance to plasma proteinase inhibitors (Figure 1.3).

Reteplase (Rapilysin® or Ecokinase®) is a single-chain non-glycosylated deletion variant consisting only of the kringle 2 and the proteinase domain of human t-PA; it contains amino acids 1–3 and 176–527 (deletion of Val^4–Glu^{175}); the Arg^{275}–Ile^{276} plasmin cleave site is maintained.[3]

In tenecteplase (TNK-rt-PA), replacement of Asn^{117} with Gln (N117Q) results in deletion of the glycosylation site in kringle 1, whereas substitution of Thr^{103} by Asn (T103N) reintroduces a glycosylation site in kringle 1, but at a different locus; these modifications substantially decrease the plasma clearance rate. In addition, the amino acids Lys^{296}–His^{297}–Arg^{298}–Arg^{299} were each replaced with Ala, which confers resistance to inhibition by PAI-1.[4] Lanoteplase is a deletion mutant of rt-PA (without the finger and growth factor domains) in which glycosylation at Asn^{117} is lacking.[5] Monteplase has a single amino acid substitution in the growth factor domain (Cys^{84}–Ser),[6] and pamiteplase has deletion of the kringle 1 domain and substitution of Arg^{275} with Glu (rendering it resistant to conversion to a two-chain molecule by plasmin).[7]

Different molecular forms of the Desmodus salivary plasminogen activator (DSPA) have been characterized. Two high M_r forms, $DSPA\alpha_1$ (43 kDa) and $DSPA\alpha_2$ (39 kDa) show about 85% homology with human t-PA, but contain neither a kringle 2 domain nor a plasmin-sensitive cleavage site. $DSPA\beta$ lacks the finger domain and $DSPA\gamma$ lacks the finger and growth factor domains.[8]

u-PA moieties

Urokinase (u-PA) is secreted as a 54-kDa single-chain molecule (scu-PA, pro-urokinase) that can be converted to a two-chain form (tcu-PA). u-PA is a serine proteinase of 411 amino acid residues, with active site triad His^{204}, Asp^{255} and Ser^{356}. The molecule contains an NH_2-terminal growth factor domain and one kringle structure homologous to the kringles of plasminogen and t-PA.[9] u-PA contains only one N-glycosylation site (at Asn^{302}), and is fucosylated at Thr^{18}. Conversion of scu-PA to tcu-PA occurs after proteolytic cleavage at position Lys^{158}–Ile^{159} by plasmin, but also by kallikrein, trypsin, cathepsin B, human T cell-associated serine proteainse-1 and thermolysin. A fully active tcu-PA derivative is obtained after additional proteolysis by plasmin at position Lys^{135}–Lys^{136}. Recombinant scu-PA (saruplase) has been expressed in *Escherichia coli* and is obtained as a 45-kDa non-glycosylated molecule.[9]

Streptokinase and derivatives

Streptokinase is a non-enzyme protein produced by several strains of hemolytic streptococci. It consists of a single polypeptide chain of 47–50 kDa with 414 amino

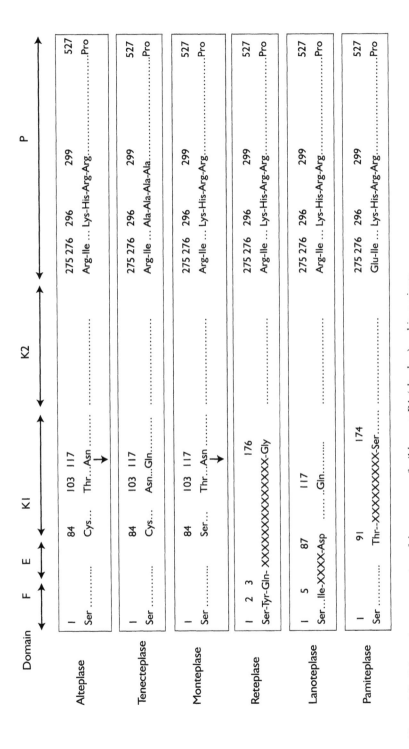

Figure 1.3 Schematic representation of the structure of wild-type t-PA (alteplase) and its variants.
F, finger domain; E, growth factor domain; K1 and K2, kringle 1 and 2; P, proteinase domain; $\downarrow$, N-linked glycosylation; XXX, deleted sequences (for more details, see text).

acid residues.[10] The region comprising residues 1–230 shows some homology with trypsin-like serine proteinases but lacks an active site serine residue.

APSAC (anistreplase, Eminase™) is an equimolar non-covalent complex between human lysine–plasminogen and streptokinase. The catalytic center is located in the COOH-terminal region of plasminogen, whereas the lysine-binding sites (with weak fibrin affinity) are contained within the NH$_2$-terminal region of the molecule. Specific acylation of the catalytic center in the complex is achieved by the use of a reversible acylating agent, p-amidinophenyl-p′-anisate.HCl. This approach should prevent premature neutralization of the agent in the bloodstream and enable its activation to proceed in a controlled and sustained manner.[11]

Staphylokinase and derivatives

Staphylokinase (Sak) is a protein of 135 amino acid residues (comprising 45 charged residues without cysteine residues or glycosylation), secreted by *Staphylococcus aureus* strains after lysogenic conversion or transformation with bacteriophages. The primary structure of Sak shows no homology with that of other plasminogen activators. Recombinant Sak is obtained by expression in *E. coli*.[12]

Staphylokinase folds into a compact ellipsoid structure in which the core of the protein is composed exclusively of hydrophobic amino acids. It is folded into a mixed five-stranded, slightly twisted β-sheet that wraps around a central α-helix and has two additional short two-stranded β-sheets opposing the central sheet.[13]

Wild-type Sak contains three immunodominant epitopes. A comprehensive site-directed mutagenesis program resulted in the identification of variants with reduced antigenicity, but maintained fibrinolytic potency and fibrin specificity, such as SakSTAR (K35A, E65Q, K74R, E80A, D82A, T90A, E99D, T101S, E108A, K109A, K130T, K135R) (code SY 161).[14] Furthermore, SY 161 with Ser in position 3 mutated into Cys, was derivatized with maleimide-substituted polyethylene glycol (P) with molecular weights of 5000 (P5), 10 000 (P10) or 20 000 (P20), and characterized *in vitro* and *in vivo* (compare below).[15]

MECHANISM OF ACTION OF FIBRINOLYTIC AGENTS

t-PA and variants

t-PA is a poor enzyme in the absence of fibrin, but the presence of fibrin strikingly enhances the activation rate of plasminogen.[16] During fibrinolysis, fibrinogen and fibrin are continuously modified by cleavage with thrombin or plasmin, yielding a diversity of reaction products.[17] Optimal stimulation of t-PA is obtained only after early plasmin cleavage in the COOH-terminal Aα-chain and the NH$_2$-terminal Bβ-chain of fibrin, yielding fragment X-polymer. Kinetic data support a mechanism in which fibrin provides a surface to which t-PA and plasminogen adsorb in a sequential and ordered way yielding a cyclic ternary complex.[16] Formation of this complex results in an enhanced affinity of t-PA for plasminogen, yielding up to three orders of magnitude higher catalytic efficiencies for plasminogen activation. This is mediated at least in part by COOH-terminal lysine residues generated by plasmin cleavage of fibrin. Plasmin formed at the fibrin surface has both its lysine-binding sites and active site occupied and is thus only slowly inactivated by α_2-antiplasmin (half-life of about 10–100 s); in contrast, free plasmin, when formed, is rapidly inhibited by α_2-antiplasmin (half-life of about 0.1 s).[18] These molecular interactions mediate the fibrin specificity of t-PA.

Reteplase has a similar plasminogenolytic activity to wild-type rt-PA in the absence of a stimulator, but its activity in the presence of a stimulator is 4-fold lower, and its binding to fibrin is 5-fold lower. Reteplase and rt-PA are inhibited by PAI-1 to a similar degree.[3]

Tenecteplase (TNK-rt-PA) has a similar ability to wild-type rt-PA for binding to fibrin, and lyses fibrin clots in a plasma milieu with enhanced fibrin specificity and delayed inhibition by PAI-1.[4] DSPAα_1 and DSPAα_2 exhibit a specific activity *in vitro* that is equal to or higher than that of rt-PA, a relative PAI-1 resistance and a greatly enhanced fibrin specificity with a strict requirement for polymeric fibrin as a cofactor.[8]

u-PA moieties

In contrast to tcu-PA, scu-PA displays very low activity toward low molecular weight chromogenic substrates; it appears, however, to have some intrinsic plasminogen activating potential, which represents $\leq 0.5\%$ of the catalytic efficiency of tcu-PA.[19] In plasma, in the absence of fibrin, scu-PA is stable and does not activate plasminogen; in the presence of a fibrin clot, scu-PA, but not tcu-PA, induces fibrin-specific clot lysis. scu-PA is an inefficient activator of plasminogen bound to internal lysine residues on intact fibrin, but has a higher activity toward plasminogen bound to newly generated COOH-terminal lysine residues on partially degraded fibrin.[20,21]

Streptokinase and derivatives

Streptokinase activates plasminogen indirectly, following a three-step mechanism.[22] In the first step, streptokinase forms an equimolar complex with plasminogen, which undergoes a conformational change resulting in the exposure of an active site in the plasminogen moiety. In the second step, this active site catalyzes the activation of plasminogen to plasmin. In a third step, plasminogen–streptokinase molecules are converted to plasmin–streptokinase complexes. The active site residues in the plasmin–streptokinase complex are the same as those in the plasmin molecule. The main differences between the enzymatic properties of both moieties are that plasmin, in contrast to its complex with streptokinase, is unable to activate plasminogen, and is rapidly neutralized by α_2-antiplasmin, which does not inhibit the complex. Since streptokinase generates free circulating plasmin when α_2-antiplasmin becomes exhausted, its use is associated with generation of a systemic lytic state.

The reversible blocking of the catalytic site by acylation (APSAC) delays the formation of plasmin but has no influence on the lysine-binding sites involved in binding of the complex to fibrin, although the affinity of plasminogen for fibrin is rather weak. Deacylation uncovers the catalytic center, which converts plasminogen to plasmin.[11]

Staphylokinase and derivatives

Sak forms a 1:1 stoichiometric complex with plasmin(ogen). It is not an enzyme, and generation of an active site in its equimolar complex with plasminogen requires conversion of plasminogen to plasmin. In plasma, in the absence of fibrin, no significant amounts of plasmin–Sak complex are generated because traces of plasmin are inhibited by α_2-antiplasmin. In the presence of fibrin, generation of the active complex is facilitated because traces of fibrin-bound plasmin are protected from α_2-antiplasmin, and inhibition of the complex at the clot surface is delayed more than 100-fold. Furthermore, Sak does not bind to a significant extent to plasminogen in circulating plasma, but binds with high affinity to plasmin and to plasminogen which is bound to partially degraded fibrin.[23] During the activation process, the 10 NH_2-terminal amino acid residues of Sak are cleaved off. With SY 161 this results in removal of the polyethylene glycol moiety.

PHARMACODYNAMICS OF FIBRINOLYTIC AGENTS

t-PA and variants

Because of its fibrin-specific mechanism of plasminogen activation, t-PA has been developed for thrombolytic therapy. Following several pilot studies with natural t-PA produced by Bowes melanoma cells, rt-PA was administered to patients with AMI.[1] It was shown to be effective and to be cleared from the circulation with an initial half-life of 4–8 min.[24] Clearance is the result of interaction with several receptor systems. Liver endothelial cells have a mannose receptor that recognizes the high mannose-type carbohydrate side-chain at Asn^{117} in the kringle 1 domain, whereas liver parenchymal cells contain a calcium-dependent receptor that interacts mainly with the growth factor domain of t-PA.[25] In addition, the low-density lipoprotein receptor-related protein (LRP), expressed in high copy number on hepatocytes, binds free t-PA and its complexes with PAI-1.[26]

Numerous clinical trials have compared the thrombolytic properties of rt-PA (alteplase, Activase®, Actilyse®) with those of other agents, culminating in the GUSTO trial and its angiographic substudy that conclusively established the potential and limitations of rt-PA for thrombolytic therapy in AMI patients.[27,28]

In the GUSTO trial, a dose of 15 mg intravenous bolus of alteplase followed by 0.75 mg/kg over 30 min (not to exceed 50 mg) and then 0.50 mg/kg over 60 min (not to exceed 35 mg) was utilized. In the COBALT trial, double bolus administration of rt-PA (50 mg given 30 min apart) was evaluated in patients with myocardial infarction.[29] Whichever regimen is used, it is important to co-administer intravenous heparin during and after alteplase treatment.

The rapid *in vivo* clearance of rt-PA, necessitating the use of large therapeutic doses, and the occurrence of bleeding complications and reocclusion, have triggered the search for improved rt-PA moieties. Mutants of rt-PA with higher fibrin specificity, more zymogenicity, slower clearance from the circulation and resistance to plasma proteinase inhibitors have been constructed (reviewed in reference 30), and are currently under investigation in pilot studies, mainly in patients with AMI. The main advantage of these newer agents appears to be their prolonged half-life, allowing bolus administration (reviewed in reference 31).

Reteplase has an initial half-life of 14–18 min. In the GUSTO-III trial, about 15 000 patients with AMI were randomly assigned to receive reteplase (two boluses of 10 million units given 30 min apart) or 100 mg alteplase over 90 min. No clinical benefit of reteplase over alteplase was demonstrated, in terms of 30-day mortality or frequency of hemorrhagic stroke, leading to the conclusion that both agents are equivalent.[32] Feasibility and timing of prehospital administration of reteplase in AMI patients is under investigation.

Tenecteplase has an initial half-life of about 20 min in AMI patients. In the TIMI-10B trial, a phase 2 efficacy trial, a single bolus of 40 mg tenecteplase yielded similar TIMI-3 flow rates at 90 min to accelerated front-loaded rt-PA, with faster and more complete reperfusion.[33] In the ASSENT-2 study (about 17 000 patients with AMI of less than 6 h) 0.53 mg/kg bolus tenecteplase yielded similar 30-day mortality and rate of intracranial bleeding to front-loaded alteplase.[34] One year after randomization, mortality rates were still similar in patients treated with tenecteplase or alteplase.[35] Furthermore, it was shown that single bolus administration of tenecteplase did not increase the risk of intracranial hemorrhage, but was associated with less non-cerebral bleeding, especially amongst high-risk patients.[36] In another substudy of ASSENT-2 the antiplatelet properties (inhibition of aggregation and function) of tenecteplase were found to be more pronounced than those of rt-PA; this may be relevant to studies on combination therapy with thrombolytic and antiplatelet agents in patients with AMI.[37] The thrombolytic properties of tenecteplase in patients with AMI have recently been reviewed in detail.[38]

With lanoteplase, given as a single bolus in the Intravenous n-PA for Treating Infarcting Myocardium Early (InTIME-2) trial (about 15 000 patients), the 30-day mortality was similar to that obtained with front-loaded alteplase, but the rate of cerebral hemorrhage was significantly increased in the lanoteplase group.[39] Following single bolus administration of lanoteplase a plasma half-life of about 35 min was observed, and at a dose of 120 kU/kg the plasminogen activator activity persisted for 6 h as compared with less than 4 h after 100 mg alteplase.[40]

Monteplase has a half-life of 23 min following bolus injection of 0.22 mg/kg.[41] In the FAST trial, the efficacy and safety of thrombolysis with monteplase and subsequent transluminal therapy for the early achievement of TIMI-3 flow were evaluated in AMI patients. The intervention resulted in significant reduction of the time to reach TIMI-3 flow as compared to thrombolysis with monteplase alone, without complications or effects on 30-day mortality. TIMI-3 flow was achieved at an earlier stage with a single bolus of monteplase as compared with an accelerated infusion of rt-PA.[42]

Pamiteplase has a half-life of 30–47 min following single bolus injection of 0.5–4 mg in human volunteers;[43] it was investigated in a dose-finding study in patients with acute myocardial infarction,[44] but no large-scale trial on safety or mortality was reported.

In several animal models of thrombolysis, DSPAα_1 (desmoteplase) had a 2.5 times higher potency and 4–8-fold slower clearance than rt-PA (for references, see in reference 30). Pilot studies have been performed in patients with AMI, but at present desmoteplase is mainly investigated in patients with stroke or pulmonary embolism.

u-PA moieties

The main mechanism of removal of u-PA from the blood is by hepatic clearance. scu-PA is taken up in the liver via a recognition site on parenchymal cells and is subsequently degraded in the lysosomes.[45] Following intravenous infusion of scu-PA in AMI patients, a biphasic disappearance was observed with initial half-life in plasma (post-infusion) of 4–8 min.[46]

With a preparation containing 160 000 IU/mg of saruplase, the dose used successfully in patients with AMI (PRIMI, Pro-urokinase in Myocardial Infarction study) was 20 mg given as a bolus and 60 mg over the next 60 min, immediately followed by an intravenous heparin infusion (20 IU/kg per h) for 72 h.[47] Early patency rate at 60 min (TIMI grade 2 and 3 flow) was significantly higher with saruplase (71.8%) than with streptokinase (48%). A 5-year follow-up of the PRIMI trial indicated a similar long-term outcome in terms of mortality and cardiovascular events in patients treated with saruplase or streptokinase, and somewhat lower reinfarction rates but higher stroke rates in the streptokinase group.[48] In the SESAM (Study in Europe with Saruplase and Alteplase in Myocardial Infarction) study, 60-min patency rates were 79.9% with saruplase versus 75.3% with alteplase, and 90-min patency rates were 79.9% versus 81.4%, respectively.[49] In the LIMITS (Liquemin in Myocardial Infarction during Thrombolysis with Saruplase) Study in AMI patients, the same dose regimen of saruplase was used, but with a prethrombolytic heparin bolus of 5000 IU and an i.v. heparin infusion for 5 days starting 30 min after completion of thrombolysis.[50] The reocclusion rates within 24–40 h were between 0.9% and 2.4% in the saruplase studies. In the PATENT (Pro-urokinase and t-PA Enhancement of Thrombolysis) trial, sequential combination of low-dose rt-PA (5–10 mg bolus) and reduced dose pro-urokinase (90 min infusion at 40 mg/h) produced a high TIMI-2 or -3 patency rate (77%), was well tolerated and was associated with a low 24-h reocclusion rate.[51]

Recombinant pro-urokinase has also been evaluated for intra-arterial administration to patients with middle cerebral artery occlusion treated within 6 h of stroke onset. The clinical efficiency and safety have been demonstrated in the PROACT I and II (Prolyse in Acute Cerebral Thromboembolism) trials.[52,53]

Streptokinase and derivatives

The elimination half-life of streptokinase in man is approximately 20 min (initial half-life of 4 min and terminal half-life of 30 min).[54] High-dose (1.5 million units), short-term (15–60 min infusion) streptokinase treatment has been routinely used in patients with acute myocardial infarction. A few days after streptokinase administration, the antistreptokinase titer rises rapidly and remains high for at least 4–6 months, during which period renewed thrombolytic treatment with streptokinase or compounds containing streptokinase is impracticable since exceedingly high doses are required to overcome the antibodies.

The activity of APSAC is controlled by the deacylation rate; the deacylation half-life in human plasma is 105–120 min.[55] In healthy volunteers, an apparent clearance half-life of 70 min was found for anistreplase, as compared to 25 min for the plasminogen–streptokinase complex formed upon administration of streptokinase alone.[54] In patients with acute myocardial infarction treated with anistreplase, half-lives of 90–112 min were reported for the plasma clearance of fibrinolytic activity.[56]

The recommended dose of anistreplase in acute myocardial infarction is 30 units (1 mg equals 1 unit and 30 mg contains approximately 1.1×10^6 units of streptokinase) to be given as a bolus injection. In aggregate, comparative studies indicate that the efficacy for coronary thrombolysis of anistreplase is comparable to or somewhat higher than intravenous streptokinase but lower than intracoronary streptokinase. Since anistreplase contains streptokinase, it causes immunization.[57]

Staphylokinase and derivatives

In patients with acute myocardial infarction, intravenous infusion of 10 mg staphylokinase over 30 min resulted in a biphasic post-infusion disappearance of staphylokinase-related antigen from plasma with a $t1/2\alpha$ of 6.3 min and a $t1/2\beta$ of 37 min, corresponding to a plasma clearance of 270 ml/min.[58,59]

Intravenous staphylokinase (10 or 20 mg), combined with heparin and aspirin, was shown to be a potent, rapidly acting and highly fibrin-selective thrombolytic agent in AMI patients.[23] The CAPTORS trial (Collaborative Angiographic Patency Trial Of Recombinant Staphylokinase) studied the optimal dose (15–45 mg) required to achieve TIMI-3 flow at 90 min with an acceptable safety profile.[60] Surprisingly, TIMI-3 patency rates were independent of the dose given.

A multicenter randomized trial compared the effects of double-bolus staphylokinase administration versus accelerated and weight-adjusted rt-PA on early coronary artery patency in patients with acute myocardial infarction.[61] Patients randomized to double-bolus staphylokinase were given 15 mg over 5 min, with a second bolus of 15 mg 30 min later. Of the patients receiving double-bolus staphylokinase, 68% had TIMI-3 flow after 90 min, versus 57% after rt-PA administration. At 24 h, TIMI perfusion grade 3 rates were 100% in the staphylokinase group, and 79% in the t-PA-treated group. The rates of hemorrhagic, mechanical and electrical complications did not significantly differ between treatment groups. Double-bolus administration of staphylokinase also preserved plasma fibrinogen, plasminogen and α_2-antiplasmin levels to a higher degree than rt-PA.

However, most patients developed high titers of neutralizing specific IgG after infusion of staphylokinase, which would predict therapeutic refractoriness upon repeated administration. Efforts have been made to reduce the immunogenicity of staphylokinase by site-directed mutagenesis and to reduce the plasma clearance by derivation with polyethylene glycol. Staphylokinase-related antigen following bolus injection of SY 161-P5, SY 161-P10 or SY 161-P20 in patients disappeared from plasma with an initial half-life of 13, 30 and 120 min and was cleared at a rate of 75, 43 and 8 ml/min, respectively, as compared to an initial half-life of 3 min and a clearance of 360 ml/min for wild-type staphylokinase.[15] Intravenous bolus injection of 5 mg of SY 161-P5 in 18 patients with AMI restored TIMI-3 flow at 60 min in 14 patients. In a multicenter dose-range finding angiographic trial (CAPTORS II), doses of 0.01 to 0.05 mg/kg SY 161-P5 yielded similar 60-min TIMI-2 or -3 patency rates to rt-PA.[62] Further studies with (pegylated) staphylokinase variants will be required to define the optimal efficacy and safety profile in patients with AMI.

The pharmacology of thrombolytic agents is summarized in Table 1.1.

CONCLUSIONS

Presently available thrombolytic agents include non-fibrin-specific plasminogen activators (streptokinase, tcu-PA, APSAC) and fibrin-specific agents (t-PA, scu-PA, staphylokinase). The clinical benefits of thrombolytic therapy in patients with acute myocardial infarction are well documented, and a close correlation between early coronary artery recanalization and clinical outcome is established. However, all available thrombolytic agents still have significant shortcomings, including the need for large therapeutic doses, limited fibrin specificity and significant associated bleeding tendency and reocclusion. As a promising new development towards improvement of thrombolytic agents, mutants and variants of tissue-type plasminogen activator have been produced with reduced plasma clerarance and lower reactivity with proteinase inhibitors and with maintained or enhanced plasminogen activator potency and/or fibrin specificity. In addition, the bacterial plasminogen activator staphylokinase has shown promise for fibrin-specific thrombolysis, although neutralizing antibodies are elicited in most patients. Pegylated staphylokinase variants have been produced with reduced immunogenicity and prolonged circulating half-life. The potential therapeutic benefit of these agents is currently being evaluated in large-scale randomized efficacy and safety studies in patients with thromboembolic diseases.

Table 1.1 Pharmacology of thrombolytic agents

Agent	M_r (kDa)	Plasma half-life/(min)	Fibrin selectivity	Inhibition by PAI-1	Dose*	Antigenicity
Alteplase	70	4–8	++	Yes	100 mg/90 min	–
Tenecteplase	70	11–20	+++	No	≈ 0.5 mg/kg bolus	–
Reteplase	39	14–18	+	Yes	2×10 MU bolus, 30 min apart	–
Lanoteplase	53.5	23–27	+	Yes	120 MU/kg bolus	–
Monteplase	68	23	++	Yes	0.22 mg/kg bolus	–
Pamiteplase	58	30–47	++	Yes	0.1 mg/kg bolus	–
Saruplase	46.5	9	±	No	80 mg/60 min	–
Staphylokinase (Sak)	16	3–6	+++	No	20 mg/30 min	++
PEG-Sak	21	15	+++	No	5 mg bolus	+
Streptokinase	47–50	25**	–	No	1.5×10^6 U/60 min	++
APSAC	≈130	70**	±	No	30 U bolus***	++

MU, million units

*Most frequently used/tested dose in patients with acute myocardial infarction

**Clearance half-life of the complex with plasminogen

***30 U APSAC contain about 1.1×10^6 U of streptokinase

REFERENCES

1. Collen D. Thrombolytic therapy. Thromb Haemost 1997; 78: 742–6

2. Pennica D, Holmes WE, Kohr WJ, et al. Cloning and expression of human tissue-type plasminogen activator cDNA in E. coli. Nature 1983; 301: 214–21

3. Kohnert U, Rudolph R, Verheijen JH, et al. Biochemical properties of the kringle 2 and protease domains are maintained in the refolded t-PA deletion variant BM 06.022. Prot Engineer 1992; 5: 93–100

4. Paoni NF, Keyt BA, Refino CJ, et al. A slow clearing, fibrin-specific, PAI-1 resistant variant of t-PA (T103N,KHRR296-299AAAA). Thromb Haemost 1993; 70: 307–12

5. Den Heijer P, Vermeer F, Ambrosioni E, et al. Evaluation of a weight-adjusted single-bolus plasminogen activator in patients with myocardial infarction: a double-blind, randomized angiographic trial of lanoteplase versus alteplase. Circulation 1998; 98: 2117–25

6. Suzuki S, Saito M, Suzuki N, et al. Thrombolytic properties of a novel modified human tissue-type plasminogen activator (E6010): a bolus injection of E6010 has equivalent potency of lysing young and aged canine coronary thrombi. J Cardiovasc Pharmacol 1991; 17: 738–46

7. Katoh M, Suzuki Y, Miyamoto T, et al. Biochemical and pharmacokinetic properties of YM866, a novel fibrinolytic agent. Thromb Haemost 1991; 65: 1193 (Abstract 1794)

8. Krätzschmar J, Haendler B, Langer G. The plasminogen activator family from the salivary gland of the vampire bat Desmodus rotundus: cloning and expression. Gene 1991; 105: 229–37

9. Holmes WE, Pennica D, Blaber M, et al. Cloning and expression of the gene for pro-urokinase in Escherichia coli. Biotechnology 1985; 3: 923–9

10. Jackson KW, Tang J. Complete amino acid sequence of streptokinase and its homology with serine proteases. Biochemistry 1982; 21: 6620–5

11. Smith RAG, Dupe RJ, English PD, Green J. Fibrinolysis with acyl-enzymes: a new approach to thrombolytic therapy. Nature 1981; 290: 505–8

12. Collen D, Zhao ZA, Holvoet P, Marynen P. Primary structure and gene structure of staphylokinase. Fibrinolysis 1992; 6: 226–31

13. Rabijns A, De Bondt HL, De Ranter C. Three-dimensional structure of staphylokinase, a plasminogen activator with therapeutic potential. Nat Struct Biol 1997; 4: 357–60

14. Laroche Y, Heymans S, Capaert S, et al. Recombinant staphylokinase variants with reduced antigenicity due to elimination of B-lymphocyte epitopes. Blood 2000; 96: 1425–32

15. Collen D, Sinnaeve P, Demarsin E, et al. Polyethylene glycol-derivatized cysteine-substitution variants of recombinant staphylokinase for single-bolus treatment of acute myocardial infarction. Circulation 2000; 102: 1766–72

16. Hoylaerts M, Rijken DC, Lijnen HR, Collen D. Kinetics of the activation of plasminogen by human tissue plasminogen activator. Role of fibrin. J Biol Chem 1982; 257: 2912–19

17. Thorsen S. The mechanism of plasminogen activation and the variability of the fibrin effector during tissue-type plasminogen activator-mediated fibrinolysis. Ann NY Acad Sci 1992; 667: 52–63

18. Collen D. On the regulation and control of fibrinolysis. Thromb Haemost 1980; 43: 77–89

19. Lijnen HR, Van Hoef B, Nelles L, Collen D. Plasminogen activation with single-chain urokinase-type plasminogen activator (scu-PA). Studies with active site mutagenized

plasminogen (Ser740→Ala) and plasmin-resistant scu-PA (Lys158→Glu). J Biol Chem 1990; 265: 5232–6

20. Liu JN, Gurewich V. Fragment E-2 from fibrin substantially enhances pro-urokinase-induced Glu-plasminogen activation. A kinetic study using the plasmin-resistant mutant pro-urokinase Ala-158-rpro-UK. Biochemistry 1992; 31: 6311–17

21. Fleury V, Lijnen HR, Anglès-Cano E. Mechanism of the enhanced intrinsic activity of single-chain urokinase-type plasminogen activator during ongoing fibrinolysis. J Biol Chem 1993; 268: 18554–9

22. Reddy KNN. Mechanism of activation of human plasminogen by streptokinase. In: Kline DL, Reddy KNN, eds. Fibrinolysis. Boca Raton, FL: CRC Press, 1980: 71–94

23. Collen D. Staphylokinase: a potent, uniquely fibrin-selective thrombolytic agent. Nat Med 1998; 4: 279–84

24. Garabedian HD, Gold HK, Leinbach RC, et al. Comparative properties of two clinical preparations of recombinant human tissue-type plasminogen activator in patients with acute myocardial infarction. J Am Coll Cardiol 1987; 9: 599–607

25. Kuiper J, Van't Hof A, Otter M, et al. Interaction of mutants of tissue-type plasminogen activator with liver cells: effect of domain deletions. Biochem J 1996; 313: 775–80

26. Orth K, Madison EL, Gething MJ, et al. Complexes of tissue-type plasminogen activator and its serpin inhibitor plasminogen-activator inhibitor type 1 are internalized by means of the low density lipoprotein receptor-related protein/alpha 2-macroglobulin receptor. Proc Natl Acad Sci USA 1992; 89: 7422–6

27. The GUSTO Investigators. An international randomized trial comparing four thrombolytic strategies for acute myocardial infarction. N Engl J Med 1993; 329: 673–82

28. GUSTO Angiographic Investigators. The effects of tissue plasminogen activator, streptokinase or both on coronary-artery patency, ventricular function, and survival after acute myocardial infarction. N Engl J Med 1993; 329: 1615–22

29. The COBALT Investigators. A comparison of continuous infusion of alteplase with double-bolus administration for acute myocardial infarction. N Engl J Med 1997; 337: 1124–30

30. Lijnen HR, Collen D. New thrombolytic strategies and agents. Hematologica 2000; 85 (Suppl 2): 106–9

31. Armstrong PW, Granger C, Van de Werf F. Bolus fibrinolysis; risk, benefit and opportunities. Circulation 2001; 103: 1171–3

32. The Gusto-III investigators. A comparison of reteplase with alteplase for acute myocardial infarction. N Engl J Med 1997; 337: 1118–23

33. Cannon CP, Gibson MC, McCabe CH, et al. TNK-tissue plasminogen activator compared with front-loaded tissue plasminogen activator in acute myocardial infarction: results of the TIMI-10B trial. Circulation 1998; 98: 2805–14

34. Assessment of the Safety and Efficacy of a New Thrombolytic (ASSENT-2) Investigators. Single-bolus tenecteplase compared with front-loaded alteplase in acute myocardial infarction: the ASSENT-2 double-blind randomised trial. Lancet 1999; 354: 716–22

35. Sinnaeve P, Alexander J, Belmans A, et al. One-year follow-up of the ASSENT-2 trial: a double-blind, randomized comparison of single-bolus tenecteplase and front-loaded alteplase in 16,949 patients with ST-elevation acute myocardial infarction. Am Heart J 2003; 146: 27–32

36. Van de Werf F, Barron HV, Armstrong PW, et al. Incidence and predictors of bleeding events after fibrinolytic therapy with fibrin-specific agents: a comparison of TNK-tPA and rt-PA. Eur Heart J 2001; 22: 2253–61

37. Serebruany VL, Malinin AI, Callahan KP, et al. Effect of tenecteplase versus alteplase on platelets during the first 3 hours of treatment for acute myocardial infarction: the Assessment of the Safety and Efficacy of a New Thrombolytic Agent (ASSENT-2) platelet substudy. Am Heart J 2003; 145: 636–42

38. Guerra DR, Karha J, Gibson CM. Safety and efficacy of tenecteplase in acute myocardial infarction. Expert Opin Pharmacother 2003; 4: 791–8

39. The InTime-II Investigators. Intravenous nPA for the treatment of infarcting myocardium early: InTime-II, a double blind comparison of single bolus lanoteplase vs accelerated alteplase for the treatment of patients with acute myocardial infarction. Eur Heart J 2000; 21: 2005–13

40. Kostis JB, Dockens RC, Thadani U, et al. Comparison of pharmacokinetics of lanoteplase and alteplase during acute myocardial infarction. Clin Pharmacokinet 2002; 41: 445–52

41. Kawai C, Yui Y, Hosada S, et al. A prospective, randomized, double-blind multicenter trial of a single bolus injection of the novel modified t-PA E6010 in the treatment of acute myocardial infarction: comparison with native t-PA. J Am Coll Cardiol 1997; 29: 1447–53

42. Nagao K, Hayashi K, Kanmatsuse K, et al. An early and complete reperfusion strategy for acute myocardial infarction using fibrinolysis and subsequent transluminal therapy – The FAST trial. Circ J 2002; 66: 576–82

43. Hashimoto K, Oikawa K, Miyamoto I. Phase I study of a novel modified t-PA. Jpn J Med Pharm Sci 1996; 36: 623–46

44. Yui Y, Haze K, Kawai C. Randomized, double-blind multicenter trial of YM866 (modified t-PA) by intravenous bolus injection in patients with acute myocardial infarction in comparison with tisokinase (native t-PA). J New Remedies Clin 1996; 45: 2175–221

45. Kuiper J, Rijken DC, de Munk GAW, van Berkel TJ. In vivo and in vitro interaction of high and low molecular weight single-chain urokinase-type plasminogen activator with rat liver cells. J Biol Chem 1992; 267: 1589–95

46. Van de Werf F, Vanhaecke J, De Geest H, et al. Coronary thrombolysis with recombinant single-chain urokinase-type plasminogen activator (rscu-PA) in patients with acute myocardial infarction. Circulation 1986; 74: 1066–70

47. PRIMI Trial Study Group. Randomised double-blind trial of recombinant pro-urokinase against streptokinase in acute myocardial infarction. Lancet 1989; 1: 863–8

48. Spiecker M, Windeler J, Vermeer F, et al. Thrombolysis with saruplase versus strepto-kinase in acute myocardial infarction: five-years results of the PRIMI trial. Am Heart J 1999; 138: 518–24

49. Bar FW, Meyer J, Vermeer F, et al. Comparison of saruplase and alteplase in acute myocardial infarction. SESAM Study Group. The Study in Europe with Saruplase and Alteplase in Myocardial Infarction. Am J Cardiol 1997; 79: 727–32

50. Tebbe U, Windeler J, Boesl I, et al., on behalf of the LIMITS Study Group. Thrombolysis with recombinant unglycosylated single-chain urokinase-type plasminogen activator (Saruplase) in acute myocardial infarction: influence on early patency rate (LIMITS Study). J Am Coll Cardiol 1995; 26: 365–73

51. Zarich SW, Kowalchuk GJ, Weaver WD, et al. Sequential combination thrombolytic therapy for acute myocardial infarction: results of the Pro-Urokinase and t-PA Enhancement of Thrombolysis (PATENT) trial. J Am Coll Cardiol 1995; 26: 374–9

52. del Zoppo GJ, Higashida RT, Furlan AJ, et al. PROACT: a phase II randomized trial of recombinant pro-urokinase by direct arterial delivery in acute middle cerebral artery stroke. PROACT Investigators. Prolyse in Acute Cerebral Thromboembolism. Stroke 1998; 29: 4–11

53. Furlan AJ, Abou-Chebi A. The role of recombinant pro-urokinase (r-pro-UK) and intra-arterial thrombolysis in acute ischaemic stroke: the PROACT trials. Prolyse in Acute Cerebral Thromboembolism. Curr Med Res Opin 2002; 18 (Suppl 2): s44–7

54. Staniforth DH, Smith RAG, Hibbs M. Streptokinase and anisoylated streptokinase plasminogen complex. Their action on haemostasis in human volunteers. Eur J Clin Pharmacol 1983; 24: 751–6

55. Ferres H, Hibbs M, Smith RAG. Deacylation studies in vitro on anisoylated plasminogen streptokinase activator complex. Drugs 1987; 33 (Suppl 3): 80–2

56. Nunn B, Esmail A, Fears R, et al. Pharmacokinetic properties of anisoylated plasminogen streptokinase activator complex and other thrombolytic agents in animals and in humans. Drugs 1987; 33 (Suppl 3): 88–92

57. Hoffmann JJML, Bonnier JJRM, de Swart JBRM, et al. Systemic effects of anisoylated plasminogen streptokinase activator complex and streptokinase therapy in acute myocardial infarction. Drugs 1987; 33 (Suppl 3): 242–6

58. Collen D, Van de Werf F. Coronary thrombolysis with recombinant staphylokinase in patients with evolving myocardial infarction. Circulation 1993; 87: 1850–3

59. Vanderschueren S, Barrios L, Kerdsinchai P, et al. A randomized trial of recombinant staphylokinase versus alteplase for coronary artery patency in acute myocardial infarction. Circulation 1995; 92: 2044–9

60. Armstrong P, Burton J, Palisaitis D, et al. Collaborative angiographic patency trial of recombinant staphylokinase (CAPTORS). Am Heart J 2000; 139: 820–3

61. Vanderschueren S, Collen D, Van de Werf F. A pilot study on bolus administration of recombinant staphylokinase for coronary artery thrombolysis. Thromb Haemost 1996; 76: 541–4

62. Armstrong PW, Burton J, Pakola S, et al., CAPTORS II Investigators. Collaborative Angiographic Patency Trial of Recombinant Staphylokinase (CAPTORS II). Am Heart J 2003; 146: 484–8

2

Prehospital triage and treatment of suspected acute myocardial infarction

Eric Boersma

TIME IS MUSCLE, AND MUSCLE IS LIFE

Experimental and clinical data support the concept that an acute myocardial infarction usually occurs as a result of a sudden thrombotic obstruction of the infarct-related coronary artery, superimposed on a ruptured atherosclerotic plaque.[1] The duration of the coronary occlusion and the extent of collateral circulation are the main determinants of infarct size in pigs, dogs, cats and other animals.[2-7] In animals with a coronary collateral circulation similar to that of humans, an occlusion persisting for 15–30 min generally does not lead to significant myocardial damage. Therefore, necrosis can be prevented provided reperfusion is achieved within this period. A small area of necrosis usually occurs with reperfusion after 45 min occlusion, while the mid-endocardial and sub-endocardial zones are still viable. Longer durations of coronary occlusion result in progressive growth of the infarction and reduction of the amount of salvageable myocardium (Figure 2.1). At 90 min the extent of cell death involves 40–50% of the area at risk; less than half of the jeopardized myocardium remains viable at that time point. Six hours after the onset of continuous ischemia the area at risk is fully infarcted, so that myocardial salvage will be minimal.

In humans, the thrombotic event frequently consists of multiple cycles of temporary occlusion and reperfusion. The degree of chest pain varies among patients, so that it is often difficult to determine the exact duration of the coronary occlusion. Nevertheless, data indicate that evolution of (enzymatically detectable) infarct size over time in humans shows a pattern similar to that in animals. In a study involving 1334 myocardial infarction patients, the cumulative release of myocardial α-hydroxybutyrate dehydrogenase during the first 72 h after infarction was comparatively small in those treated within 1 h from onset of symptoms (Figure 2.2).[8] A very steep increase in the rate of enzyme release was noted between 1 and 2 h of treatment delay, whereas the increase was relatively small thereafter.

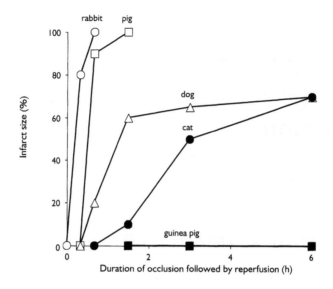

Figure 2.1 Development of infarct size as a percentage of the infarct size that would occur if the coronary artery were permanently occluded in various animal species. Figure adapted from reference 3 and modified.

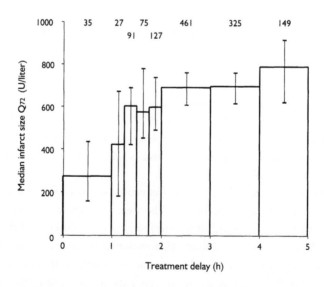

Figure 2.2 Effect of delay of fibrinolytic treatment on infarct size. Numbers above columns are numbers of patients. Columns represent mean values; vertical bars represent 95% confidence intervals. Q_{72}, cumulative activity of myocardial α-hydroxybutyrate dehydrogenase released per liter of plasma during the first 24 h after acute myocardial infarction. Figure adapted from reference 8 and modified.

Treatment delay and the effectiveness of fibrinolytic therapy

The value of fibrinolytic therapy in patients with evolving myocardial infarction is well documented. Timely fibrinolytic therapy interrupts the process of evolving myocardial necrosis, which results in salvage of viable myocardium, preservation of left ventricular function and, consequently, improved survival. A meta-analysis of large randomized trials that compared fibrinolytic therapy with control (including almost 60 000 patients) showed an absolute mortality reduction of about 30 per 1000 patients presenting within 6 h, and of about 20 per 1000 patients presenting between 6 and 12 h from onset of symptoms.[9] A more detailed analysis of the relation between treatment delay and treatment effect, which also included data from smaller trials, indicated that the mortality reduction by fibrinolytic therapy was greatest among patients presenting within 1 h from symptom onset.[10] The proportional mortality reduction in this group was as high as 50% (Figure 2.3), whereas the absolute mortality reduction was estimated at 65 per 1000 patients treated (Figure 2.4). Fibrinolytic treatment that is initiated within 2 h results in a significantly higher proportional mortality reduction than later treatment (45% versus 20%), indicating that most benefit of fibrinolysis can be obtained during the

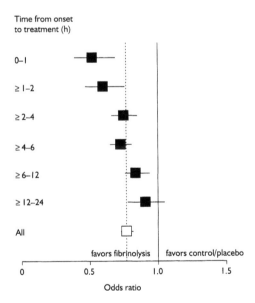

Figure 2.3 Proportional effect of fibrinolytic therapy on 35-day mortality according to treatment delay. Data are derived from all 22 trials conducted between 1983 and 1993 that included at least 100 patients who were randomized between fibrinolytic therapy or control. Odds ratios are significantly different over the six groups (Breslow-Day test, $p = 0.001$). Figure adapted from reference 10 and modified.

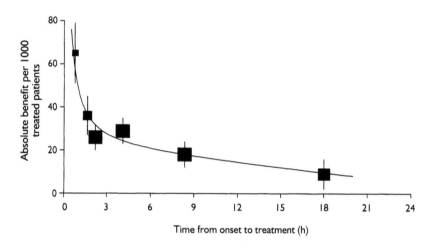

Figure 2.4 Absolute 35-day mortality reduction versus treatment delay. The regression line is fitted within data that are derived from all 22 trials conducted between 1983 and 1993 that included at least 100 patients who were randomized between fibrinolytic therapy or control. Black squares: average effects in six time-to-treatment groups (the areas of these squares are inversely proportional to the variance of absolute benefit described).
Figure adapted from reference 10 and modified.

ongoing process of myocardial cell death. Therefore, to realize the full potential of the life-saving effects of fibrinolytic therapy, treatment should be initiated as soon as possible after symptom onset, preferably within the first 1–2 h. Unfortunately, to date only a minority of myocardial infarction patients (5–10%) receive such early fibrinolysis.

Treatment delay and the effectiveness of primary percutaneous coronary intervention

As we have seen, timing of reperfusion therapy is an important determinant of the end result. Additional factors are adequate coronary blood flow restoration and the prevention of coronary reocclusion. Recent studies have shown that fibrinolytic treatment is capable of restoring coronary patency in 55–80% of cases, depending on the fibrinolytic agent used.[11] Thus, coronary reperfusion does not occur in 20–45% of patients. In addition, 5–10% of patients experience an early reocclusion, whereas 30% experience late occlusion.[12,13] An alternative approach to reopen the occluded coronary artery is to perform a primary percutaneous coronary intervention (PPCI), which is known to have a success rate of 95–99%.[14] A meta-analysis of randomized trials that compared PPCI with fibrinolysis demonstrated a 30% proportional 30-day mortality reduction in favor of the mechanical approach, whereas the absolute mortality reduction was estimated at 21 per 1000 patients treated.[15] It has been repeatedly reported that the effectiveness of PPCI is time-dependent.[16–18] In a large observational study of 27 080 patients treated by PPCI, increased mortality rates were observed after door-to-balloon times exceeding 120 min (Figure 2.5).[18] Furthermore, data from randomized trials indicate that the proportional mortality reduction of PPCI over fibrinolysis is dependent on the additional treatment delay that is introduced by the invasive approach. In particular, PPCI is associated with a 67% reduction in 30-day mortality in clinical environments with a PPCI-related delay that is limited to a maximum of 35 min, and with a 28% reduction in settings with longer PPCI-related delays (Figure 2.6).[19] The absolute mortality reduction can be estimated at 54 and 26 per 1000 patients undergoing PPCI, respectively. Thus, similar to fibrinolysis, increasing treatment delays importantly diminish the life-saving effects of PPCI.

TREATMENT DELAY IN CLINICAL PRACTICE, AND THE NEED FOR PREHOSPITAL TRIAGE AND THERAPY

The time that expires between the onset of chest pain, which is supposed to coincide with the coronary obstruction, and the initiation of reperfusion therapy consists of three main components. First, the patient needs time to recognize the cardiac nature and severity of the problems, and to seek medical help. Unfortunately, most patients

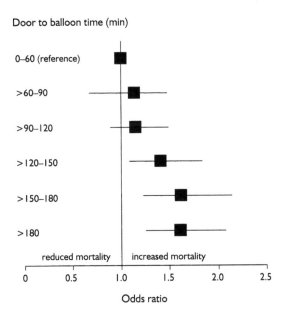

Figure 2.5 Multivariably adjusted relationship between door-to-balloon time and mortality in 27 080 patients undergoing primary percutaneous coronary intervention.
Figure adapted from reference 18 and modified.

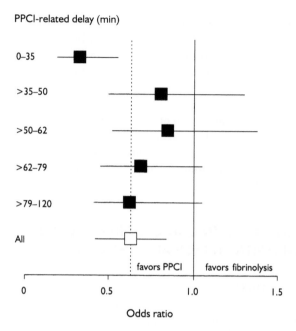

Figure 2.6 Proportional effect of primary percutaneous coronary intervention (PPCI) on 30-day mortality, relative to fibrinolysis, according to PPCI-related delay. Data are derived from randomized trials conducted between 1990 and 2003 that included at least 50 patients who were randomized between PPCI and fibrinolytic therapy. Odds ratios are adjusted for selected baseline characteristics. PPCI-related delay is defined as the hospital-specific difference between the median time from randomization to the first balloon inflation (in those undergoing PPCI) and the median time from randomization to the commencement of fibrinolysis (in those receiving such therapy).
Figure adapted from reference 19 and modified.

fail to react rapidly to symptoms. Data from (inter)national registries of myocardial infarctions in the USA and in Europe indicate that about 50% of patients who are eligible for reperfusion therapy do not report their symptoms within 3 h.[20,21] Another 25% do not arrive at the hospital emergency department until 6 h or later, including 10% who arrive 12 h or later, a period in which reperfusion therapy has lost most of its life-saving capacity.

The second component of total treatment delay is the time needed for transportation to the hospital. Depending on the local infrastructure, the distance to the nearest hospital and the hour of the day (traffic jam), the transport delay may vary considerably.[22–24] Usually it takes 10–15 min before arrival of the ambulance at the patient's home. Another 10–15 min is needed for preparation, and again another 10–15 min for the actual transport.

The third component of treatment delay is the time needed inside the hospital for nursing, initial evaluation by an emergency room physician, ECG recording and interpretation, laboratory testing, further evaluation by an experienced staff cardiologist, and transport from the emergency room to the coronary care unit or the catheterization laboratory where therapy is subsequently initiated. Data from a broad spectrum of European clinical practices demonstrate that the time needed for in-hospital decision making is considerable.[21] In patients who were selected for fibrinolysis, the median time from arrival at the emergency room to the commencement of therapy was 59 min, whereas treatment guidelines recommend that such door-to-needle times should preferably be shorter than 20 min.[25] In patients selected for PPCI, the median door-to-balloon time was as large as 93 min. Available data from other parts of the world show similar worrisome results.

One might expect that the increasing literature on the importance of early reperfusion therapy in acute myocardial infarction would have resulted in decreasing treatment delays over recent years. This, however, seems not to be the case. The mean delay from onset of symptoms to the initiation of fibrinolytic therapy in mega-trials of myocardial infarction patients (with similar inclusion criteria) has hardly changed since the beginning of the 1990s (Figure 2.7). In fact, treatment delays slightly increased since that time, with a mean value of 165 min in GUSTO-1 (1993) and 198 min in HERO-2 (2001).[26,27]

These results can be improved by a treatment strategy that aims at diagnosis and triage prior to hospital admission, using 12-lead electrocardiography.[28] In such a system, after myocardial infarction is confirmed, immediate, prehospital fibrinolytic

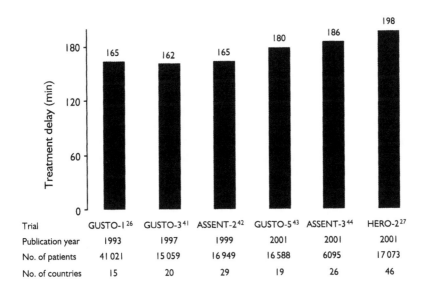

Figure 2.7 Mean time from symptom onset to fibrinolytic treatment in recent mega-trials of myocardial infarction patients. All trials randomized patients within 6 h from onset of symptoms.

therapy can be installed, or the patient can be directly transported to a catheterization laboratory, which will be prepared before arrival of the patient. Several investigations have indicated that this approach may result in a reduction of the total ischemic time by approximately 1 h, regardless of the mode of reperfusion therapy.[22–24,29]

PREHOSPITAL TRIAGE AND FIBRINOLYTIC THERAPY

Randomized trials of prehospital versus in-hospital fibrinolysis

There are eight randomized trials that have compared prehospital with in-hospital fibrinolytic therapy.[22–24,30–34] Although most of these studies were too small to show statistical significance, together they provide compelling evidence that prehospital fibrinolysis is feasible, safe and effective, on the understanding that conditions are fulfilled with regard to a proper diagnosis and with regard to (relative) contra-indications.

The European Myocardial Infarction Project (EMIP) is the largest such trial. EMIP was undertaken during 1988–1992 in 163 cardiological practices in 15 European countries and Canada.[22] Patients with chest pain suggestive of myocardial infarction and lasting for at least 30 min, or pain lasting for less than 30 min but still present and not responsive to nitrates, who were seen within 6 h from the onset of symptoms were eligible if the ECG confirmed the diagnosis of myocardial infarction. Classical electrocardiographic requirements were applied: ST segment elevation ≥1 mm in ≥2 limb leads and/or elevation ≥2 mm in ≥2 precordial leads. Excluded were patients who were at increased risk of bleeding complications (Table 2.1), and patients who were known or suspected to be pregnant. There was no upper age limit. Eligible patients who gave their consent to participate were randomly (and double-blind) assigned to immediate fibrinolytic therapy (anistreplase) followed by placebo in the hospital, or placebo before admission followed by anistreplase in the hospital. Prehospital screening, diagnosis (including ECG interpretation) and initiation of study medication was performed by ambulance attendants, nurses and accompanying physicians.

The primary study endpoint was death from all causes by 30 days. According to the design, 10 000 patients should have been randomized to detect a 15% reduction in the primary endpoint in favor of prehospital fibrinolysis, but the trial was terminated prematurely because of lack of funding. Finally, 5469 patients were enrolled. The median time from symptom onset to treatment in patients randomized to prehospital fibrinolysis was 130 min, compared to 190 min in the in-hospital group. The median time gained with prehospital treatment was 55 min. The diagnosis of myocardial infarction was confirmed in hospital in 90% of patients. Another 7% of patients had an acute coronary syndrome, but myocardial infarction could not be confirmed. Two per cent of patients were diagnosed with non-cardiac disease. Twenty-one patients (0.4%) had pericarditis. The incidence of ventricular

Table 2.1 Inclusion criteria and exclusion criteria that are applied in three major randomized clinical trials of prehospital versus in-hospital fibrinolysis

	EMIP	MITI	GREAT
Inclusion criteria			
Minimal duration of symptoms	30 min	–	20 min
Maximal duration of symptoms	6 h	6 h	4 h
No relief by nitroglycerin	X	–	–
ECG findings	X	X	–
Exclusion criteria			
Cardiac massage	X	–	X
Blood pressure	>200/120	>180/120	>200/-
Known bleeding disorder	X	–	X
Pregnancy/menstruation	X	–	X
Use of oral anticoagulants	X	–	X
Previous thrombolysis	–	–	X
History of stroke	X	X	X
Recent history of			
major trauma	X	X	X
surgery	X	X	X
percutaneous coronary intervention	X	–	–
gastroduodenal ulcer or blood loss	X	–	X

EMIP, European Myocardial Infarction Project (reference 22); MITI, Myocardial Infarction Triage and Intervention trial (reference 23); GREAT, Grampian Region Early Anistreplase Trial (reference 24)

fibrillation, shock and symptomatic hypotension during transportation was higher in patients randomized to prehospital fibrinolysis, but patients randomized to in-hospital treatment had a higher incidence of these complications during hospital stay (Table 2.2). As a result, there was no difference in the overall incidence between the two groups. Thirty-day mortality was 9.7% in patients randomized to prehospital fibrinolysis and 11.1% in in-hospital fibrinolysis, implying a 13% relative mortality reduction, and a 1.4% absolute mortality reduction.

The Myocardial Infarction Triage and Intervention (MITI) trial was performed during 1989–1991, and involved 19 hospitals in the area of Seattle, WA, USA.[23] Patients aged 75 years or younger who had symptoms suggestive of acute myocardial infarction, chest pain for less than 6 h and no risk factors for serious bleeding (Table 2.1) were further evaluated for inclusion in the trial. A 12-lead ECG was derived by a paramedic, using a portable, computer-interpreted ECG system (Marquette Electronics), and subsequently transmitted to the emergency department of the paramedic base hospital. A physician in the emergency department reviewed the clinical and ECG findings, and made the final treatment decision. Patients who consented were randomly allocated to receive either prehospital or in-hospital fibrinolytic (alteplase) treatment. No placebo was given to patients randomized to

Table 2.2 Major complications according to allocated treatment arm in three randomized clinical trials of prehospital versus in-hospital fibrinolysis

	EMIP		MITI		GREAT	
	Pre	In	Pre	In	Pre	In
Number	2750	2719	163	148	175	185
Prehospital						
Death	1.3	0.9	1.8	3.4	–	–
Ventricular fibrillation	2.5	1.6	–	–	–	–
Cardiac arrest	1.6	1.2	0	2.7	< 1	< 1
Pulmonary edema	2.3	2.3	–	–	12	
Shock	6.3	3.9	1.2	1.4	3	
Stroke	0.1	0	0	0	–	–
In-hospital						
Death	8.4	10.2	4.9	8.1	–	–
Ventricular fibrillation	11.1	13.9	–	–	–	–
Cardiac arrest	12.0	15.0	1.2	2.0	–	–
Pulmonary edema	23.0	24.9			–	–
Shock	24.6	26.5	–	–	–	–
Stroke	3.0	3.0	0.6	0.6	–	–
Total						
Death	9.7	11.1	6.7	11.5	5.3	11.9
Ventricular fibrillation	13.6	15.5	–	–	–	–
Cardiac arrest	13.6	16.2	1.2	4.7	–	–
Pulmonary edema	25.3	27.2			–	–
Shock	30.9	30.4	–	–	–	–
Stroke	3.1	3.0	0.6	0.6	2.3	1.1

EMIP, European Myocardial Infarction Project (reference 22); MITI, Myocardial Infarction Triage and Intervention trial (reference 23); GREAT, Grampian Region Early Anistreplase Trial (reference 24); Pre, randomized to prehospital fibrinolytic treatment; In, randomized to in-hospital fibrinolytic treatment

in-hospital treatment. The primary endpoint of the trial was a ranked composite score that combined death, stroke, major bleeding and infarct size.

MITI enrolled 360 patients. The median time from symptom onset to treatment was 77 min for the patients allocated to prehospital treatment and 110 min for those allocated to in-hospital treatment. The median time gained with prehospital treatment was 33 min. Myocardial infarction was confirmed in 98% of patients. One per cent of patients had no enzyme elevation, and were diagnosed with unstable angina. One patient (0.3%) had pericarditis. The composite outcome score was similar for both arms of the trial. Mortality rates were 5.7% and 8.1% in patients randomized to prehospital and in-hospital treatment, respectively.

The Grampian Region Early Anistreplase Trial (GREAT), which was undertaken during 1988–1991, involved 29 rural general practices in the region of

Grampian, Scotland.[24] These practices are located in small villages at a distance of 16–62 miles from Aberdeen, the closest city with adequate hospital facilities. Entry to the trial was a strong clinical suspicion of acute myocardial infarction by the general practitioner. Symptoms suggestive of myocardial infarction had to have been present for at least 20 min, but no longer than 4 h (because, for ethical reasons, it had to be possible for the patients to get to Aberdeen within 6 h after symptom onset). The general practitioner was equipped with an electrocardiograph and he was required to record an ECG. However, no formal ECG criteria were applied for study entry. Excluded were patients with a suspected high risk of major bleeding complications (Table 2.1). Patients who agreed to participate were randomly assigned to immediate fibrinolytic therapy (anistreplase) followed by placebo in the hospital, or placebo before admission followed by anistreplase in the hospital. Randomization was double blind. The primary endpoint of the trial was in accordance with the main purpose: to study the feasibility and safety of prehospital fibrinolytic therapy. Efficacy (i.e. mortality reduction) was a secondary endpoint.

Altogether 311 patients participated in GREAT. The median times from symptom onset to home and hospital treatment were 105 and 240 min, respectively. This difference was apparently larger than in EMIP and MITI, and can partly be explained by the large distance from the Grampian region to Aberdeen: the journey time was estimated at approximately 45 min. However, the in-hospital delays (door-to-needle time) were also considerable: about 90 min. The proportion of trial patients with a final, hospital discharge diagnosis of myocardial infarction was 78%, importantly lower than in EMIP and MITI. Eleven per cent of patients were classified with ischemic heart disease (but no infarction), whereas another 9% had a specific chest pain. It should be realized in this respect, that in GREAT no expert support was given to general practitioners for the interpretation of the qualifying ECG. Inadequate interpretation of ECGs results in a relatively low specificity of the diagnostic 'system'. Hospital discharge mortality rates were 6.7% and 11.5% in patients allocated to prehospital and in-hospital fibrinolytic treatment, respectively.

In summary, an apparent reduction in treatment delay can be reached if the diagnosis of myocardial infarction and subsequent initiation of fibrinolytic therapy can be displaced from the hospital to the patient's home. More importantly, the strategy of prehospital triage and treatment enables fibrinolytic treatment within the first 'golden' hour in a considerable proportion of patients. In the combined data of all randomized trials of prehospital versus in-hospital fibrinolysis a 1-h time gain was noted: the median delays were 125 and 186 min, respectively. This 1-h earlier treatment was associated with a benefit of approximately 20 lives per 1000 patients treated (Figure 2.8). Indeed, it is a paying option to bring the treatment to the patient.

Benefits and risks in prehospital fibrinolysis

The safety of prehospital fibrinolysis strongly depends on the possibilities of correct diagnosis in the prehospital setting. Because of the (albeit moderate) risk of severe, life-threatening bleeding complications associated with fibrinolytic agents,

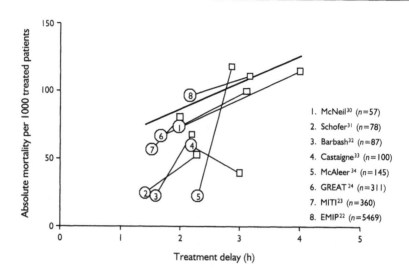

Figure 2.8 Mortality at 35 days in randomized studies comparing prehospital (circles) with in-hospital (squares) fibrinolytic therapy. All trials (except Castaigne) showed a trend favoring prehospital fibrinolysis. The regression line (bold, weighted by the number of patients included in the mortality result) was mainly determined by the EMIP study.
Figure adapted from reference 10 and modified.

inappropriate treatment should be avoided in patients with suggestive symptoms, but without developing an infarction. A correctly interpreted ECG is essential in this respect (remember the GREAT results). The occurrence of ST segment deviation (ST segment elevation and concomitant depression) on the ECG is the most specific electrocardiographic measure for confirmation of evolving myocardial infarction.[35] The percentage of myocardial infarctions to be confirmed (sensitivity) and of non-infarctions to be excluded (specificity) is related to the selected thresholds for ST deviation. The choice of these thresholds for prehospital fibrinolysis is arbitrary and depends on the perceived benefits of appropriate treatment and risks of inappropriate treatment. Figure 2.9 demonstrates the sensitivity and specificity for myocardial infarction in relation to thresholds of ST deviation as observed in a study of 1072 consecutive patients presenting within 6 h from the onset of chest pain suggestive of acute cardiac pathology.[36] These patients were transported by the ambulance service in the region of Rotterdam, The Netherlands. Ambulance nurses derived an ECG prior to hospital admission. Note that the classical criteria for in-hospital electrocardiographic confirmation of evolving myocardial infarction (ST segment elevation ≥ 1 mm in ≥ 2 limb leads and/or elevation ≥ 2 mm in ≥ 2 precordial leads) were satisfied in 49 out of 701 patients without a final diagnosis of myocardial infarction, implying a specificity of 93% of the ECG in this context. Indeed, myocardial infarction cannot be ruled out with 100% certainty in the time period during which fibrinolytic therapy is most effective.

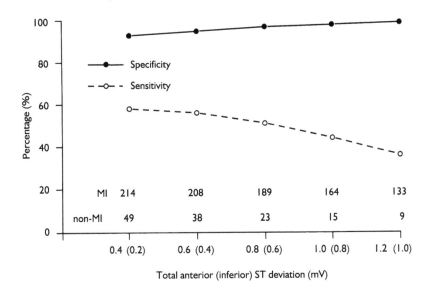

Figure 2.9 Sensitivity and specificity in confirmation of myocardial infarction (MI) at several thresholds of ST deviation on the presenting electrocardiograms. All 263 (214 + 49) patients in this figure met the classical criteria for in-hospital confirmation of infarction (≥ 2 leads of V1–V6 show ≥ 0.2 mV ST elevation or ≥ 2 leads of II, III, aVF show ≥ 0.1 mV ST elevation). ST deviation is defined as: (a) in case of anterior ST elevation: the total sum of ST elevation in V1–V6 plus ST depression in II, III, aVF and (b) otherwise (said to be inferior): the total sum of ST elevation in I, II, III, aVF, aVL, V5, V6 plus ST depression in V1–V4. Figure adapted from reference 25 and modified.

As outlined above, in Western Europe and the USA prehospital initiation of fibrinolytic treatment reduces the call-to-needle time by about 1 h compared to in-hospital therapy. The gain of earlier therapy is time-dependent (Figures 2.3 and 2.4). The average gain per hour of earlier treatment is approximately 60, 10 and 2 lives saved per 1000 treated patients in the respective 0–1 h, > 1–3 h and > 3–6 h intervals after onset of symptoms. If prehospital fibrinolysis were restricted to patients presenting within 6 h, on average, mortality reduction in definite myocardial infarction patients – the benefit of a prehospital fibrinolysis program – could reliably be estimated at 10–20 lives saved per 1000 treated. In some patients an intracranial bleeding may occur as a consequence of fibrinolytic therapy, which will lead to death in more than half of the cases and to severe disability in another quarter.[37] The risk for intracranial hemorrhage can be estimated at 5–10 per 1000 patients treated.[9,37] In patients with evolving myocardial infarction this risk is partly compensated by a reduction of the risk for embolic stroke (strokes of any type occur in approximately 4–8 per 1000 treated patients).[9,37] Moreover, the expected mortality reduction far exceeds the expected risk of intracranial hemorrhage.[9] However, in patients without infarction who (erroneously) receive fibrinolytic therapy the benefits are absent, while the bleeding risk prevails. Hence, the risk of a prehospital fibrinolysis program can be estimated at 5–10 intracranial bleeding complications per 1000 treated non-infarctions. Figure 2.10 presents the expected benefit/risk ratio at several thresholds of ST deviation. In the above-mentioned series of 1072 patients, for each four patients with a confirmed infarction who met the classical ST thresholds one patient without confirmed infarction did so, resulting in a benefit/risk ratio of 4–17.[36] This ratio can be improved by introducing additional criteria for total ST deviation, or by using stricter criteria for ST elevation. Although the question of the optimal ratio between benefits and risks in prehospital fibrinolysis cannot be answered unambiguously, these data may be of help in making rational choices in clinical practice. It should be realized in this respect that a relatively high benefit/risk ratio will result in a relatively high net benefit (estimated benefit minus risk; interpretation: the additional number of lives saved by prehospital treatment without additional cerebral complications) per patients treated, but in a relatively low net benefit per patients screened.

The Dutch experience

In 1988 a program for prehospital triage and fibrinolytic treatment was initiated in the Rotterdam area of The Netherlands.[38–40] Table 2.3 shows the inclusion and exclusion criteria for eligibility for prehospital fibrinolysis according to this

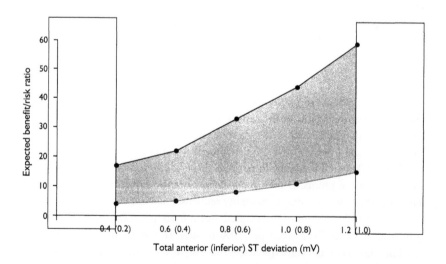

Total anterior (inferior) ST deviation (mV)

Figure 2.10 Expected benefit/risk ratio at several thresholds of ST-deviation on the presenting electrocardiograms. Only the 263 patients who met the classical in-hospital criteria (Figure 2.9) for confirmation of infarction are potential candidates for prehospital fibrinolysis. These patients contribute to the benefit/risk estimations. See Figure 2.9 for definition of ST deviation.

Figure adapted from reference 25 and modified.

Table 2.3 Main inclusion and exclusion criteria for prehospital fibrinolytic treatment according to the REPAIR program

	Criteria
Inclusion criteria	
1988 initial	chest pain suggestive of myocardial infarction, existing for ≤3 h; pain not responsive to nitroglycerin; upper age limit 70 years; for women: lower age limit 55 years (to exclude potential pregnancy)
1991 modification	chest pain suggestive of myocardial infarction, existing for ≤6 h; upper age limit 75 years; lower age limit for women dropped, but pregnancy remains an exclusion criterion
1996 modification	upper age limit 80 years
Exclusion criteria	
1988 initial	cardiopulmonary resuscitation; low consciousness; paresis or paralysis; history of stroke; uncontrolled hypertension; use of oral anticoagulants; severe trauma; recent history of blood loss; surgery within past 3 months
1991 modification	pregnancy; use of oral anticoagulants allowed; hypersensitivity to streptokinase
Electrocardiographic criteria	
1988 initial	≥3 mm ST elevation in ≥2 precordial leads OR ≥2 mm ST elevation in ≥2 limb leads; total sum of ST deviation ≥10 mm
1996 modification	≥2 mm ST elevation in ≥2 precordial leads AND ≥3 mm ST elevation in ≥1 precordial leads; total sum of ST deviation ≥6 (8) mm in case of age ≤70 (80) years OR ≥1 mm ST elevation in ≥2 limb leads AND ≥2 mm ST elevation in ≥1 limb leads; total sum of ST deviation ≥4 (6) mm in case of age ≤70 (80) years
2001 modification	total sum of ST deviation ≥15 mm: eligible for primary percutaneous coronary intervention

REPerfusion in Acute Infarction Rotterdam (REPAIR) program. In case of a suspected acute myocardial infarction the general practitioner or, in their absence, the ambulance nurse applies a short questionnaire. A portable device equipped with a computer algorithm acquires a standard 12-lead simultaneous ECG. If the device detects a major evolving myocardial infarction and the questionnaire confirms patient eligibility, the ambulance nurse initiates fibrinolytic therapy, and the crew will transport the patient to the hospital.

From June 1988 to June 2000 a total of 1487 patients received fibrinolytic treatment according to the REPAIR protocol. Of all patients 56%, 80% and 90% notified the emergency service within 1, 2 and 3 h, respectively. In nine patients (0.6%) prehospital fibrinolytic treatment was initiated whereas the diagnosed myocardial infarction could not be confirmed during hospital admission. One of these patients suffered a non-fatal hemorrhagic stroke. Two patients died during transportation, and ventricular fibrillation occurred in 40 patients (2.7%), all of whom were successfully resuscitated. No major hemorrhagic complications occurred during transportation. Mortality after 30 days, 1, 5 and 10 years was 4.9%, 7.3%, 16.2% and 30.1%, respectively. These results are highly motivating: note that 30-day and 1-year survival in recent clinical trials of myocardial infarction patients are in the range of 5.5–7% and 9–11%, respectively.[26,27,41–44] Patients treated within 2 h had a significantly lower mortality rate than those treated within 2–6 h from symptom onset (Figure 2.11), which again emphasized the importance of very early treatment. The difference remained after adjustment for age and other clinical variables.

The REPAIR program was set out to evaluate the safety and feasibility of prehospital fibrinolytic treatment in the municipal area of Rotterdam. The positive outcome of this project has prompted its continuation and integration into routine care of the Rotterdam ambulance emergency service. To date, approximately 10% of myocardial infarction patients in the region of Rotterdam receive fibrinolytic therapy before hospital admission according to the REPAIR protocol.

Another aspect of very early lysis of the intracoronary thrombus is that the infarct process can be aborted at a stage at which irreversible myocardial damage has not yet occurred. Lamfers et al. defined an aborted infarction by fibrinolytic treatment as follows: (1) a patient has chest pain and ECG changes suggestive of transmural ischemia; (2) the cumulative sum of ST segment elevation and depression decreased to < 50% within 2 h of treatment; and (3) CK-MB elevations remained below twice the upper limit of normal.[45] In a series of 224 myocardial infarction patients who were treated before hospital admission according to the Nijmegen prehospital treatment program 13% fulfilled these criteria, as compared to 4% in a comparable series of 266 patients who received in-hospital treatment.[45] Thus prehospital fibrinolysis is associated with a higher (order of magnitude: 3-fold) proportion of patients with aborted infarction than in-hospital treatment. The need to start treatment before hospital admission is sometimes questioned by cardiologists who argue that transporting times in their region are short, whereas in their practice fibrinolytic therapy will be applied very early after hospital arrival. For this time we pass over the fact that physicians tend to have an optimistic view on their own

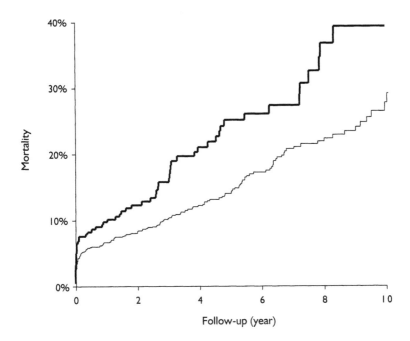

Figure 2.11 Long-term follow-up of the 1487 patients treated according to the REPAIR protocol. The thin line represents patients treated within 2 h from onset of symptoms; the bold line represents patients treated between 2 and 6 h.
Figure adapted from reference 29 and modified.

practices (see the registries data as presented above). Here is the ultimate test of this critical assertion: just count the number of aborted infarctions in your practice.

PREHOSPITAL TRIAGE AND PRIMARY PERCUTANEOUS CORONARY INTERVENTION

Only a minority of myocardial infarction patients present directly to hospitals that are adequately equipped to perform PPCI. The vast majority of patients present to the emergency ambulance service or to a hospital without angioplasty facilities. Hence, in patients selected for PPCI, additional transportation to an interventional catheterization laboratory is often necessary. It is true that this can be organized safely.[46,47] Also, PPCI remains superior to fibrinolysis even when patients are transferred to an angioplasty center.[48] Nevertheless, the additional time delay will offset part of the lifesaving potential of PPCI (Figures 2.5 and 2.6).

Part of the PPCI-related time delay can be regained by a triage system that enables myocardial infarction diagnosis prior to hospital admission, in the ambulance. As soon as a myocardial infarction is diagnosed, immediate transfer to the nearest PPCI center can be effected, while avoiding admission to a hospital without appropriate facilities. In the meantime the catheterization laboratory and the personnel can be prepared. The Pre-Hospital Infarction Angioplasty Triage (PHIAT) protocol was designed to study the feasibility of such an approach in the larger region of Zwolle, The Netherlands.[49] Myocardial infarction was diagnosed by ambulance personnel, using a portable 12-lead ECG device equipped with a dedicated computer algorithm, similar to REPAIR. Patients who were immediately transported to the PPCI center, which was located in the inner city of Zwolle, had an important 50-min shorter total ischemic time compared to patients who were initially presented to the emergency room of another hospital and then transported to the PPCI center (mean values 172 versus 220 min, respectively).[29] Even more impressive results have been obtained in the rural area of Aarhus in Denmark.[50] In that region, prehospital diagnosis was established with the use of telemedicine, by ambulance physicians, or by general practitioners. The median time from ambulance call to first balloon inflation was 81 min shorter in patients who were directly transported to a PPCI center as compared to those who were diagnosed at a local hospital (median values 87 versus 168 min, respectively).

Facilitated percutaneous coronary intervention

Facilitated PCI is a strategy of planned immediate PCI after an initial pharmacological regimen, including a fibrinolytic agent (reduced doses) or a glycoprotein (GP) IIb/IIIa inhibitor. It has been argued that such pharmacological facilitation may improve outcome, specifically in patients who are being transferred to the catheterization laboratory. PCI performed as a matter of policy immediately after fibrinolytic therapy, in order to enhance reperfusion or reduce the risk of reocclusion, has proved disappointing in a number of earlier trials, which all showed a tendency to an increased risk of complications and death. However, increased experience and the availability of stents have made PCI following pharmacological intervention safer. In the randomized trials that have been conducted to date pretreatment with a fibrinolytic agent resulted in improved preprocedural coronary patency, whereas there was no evidence of an excess bleeding risk.[51–53] However, these trials did not demonstrate any benefit in reducing infarct size or improving outcomes. Additional trials that evaluate the efficacy and safety of pretreatment with a reduced dose of a fibrinolytic agent are currently underway.

The use of GP IIb/IIIa inhibitors in ST elevation patients undergoing percutaneous intervention inhibits platelet aggregation at the site of plaque rupture and procedure-induced injury, potentially improving the clinical outcome. A total of six randomized trials of abciximab versus control therapy in patients undergoing PPCI (with or without stenting) examined this hypothesis.[54–59] In these trials, abciximab was associated with a non-significant trend toward reduction in mortality and myocardial reinfarction at 30-day follow-up compared with control therapy. Since these results are compatible with the benefit of GP IIb/IIIa inhibitors as observed in other PCI studies,[60] the medical community has accepted abciximab as a useful pharmacological co-therapy in patients undergoing PPCI. In one of the smaller randomized trials of GP IIb/IIIa inhibitors in PPCI, called ADMIRAL, the magnitude of the drug effect was considerably higher in patients in whom study medication was commenced in the ambulance, prior to arrival in the catheterization laboratory, compared with the remaining patients.[55] This observation was the catalyst for another six randomized PPCI trials that compared early administration of GP IIb/IIIa inhibitors, outside the catheterization laboratory (in the largest of these studies patients were randomized and treated in the ambulance),[61] versus delayed administration. Altogether in these trials, early administration of GP IIb/IIIa inhibitors was associated with an increased proportion of patients with adequate blood flow (TIMI grade 3) through the target vessel as observed on the initial angiogram.[62] The superior coronary flow did not translate into reduced mortality or non-fatal re-infarction, but it has to be acknowledged that trials were underpowered to demonstrate significant differences in these endpoints. Nevertheless, these findings are supportive of a strategy of facilitated PPCI by a GP IIb/IIIa inhibitor. Randomized trials evaluating the clinical efficacy and safety of this strategy are currently being conducted.

FIBRINOLYSIS OR PPCI? TIME MATTERS!

The discussion on whether or not PPCI or fibrinolysis should be the preferred treatment option for patients presenting with ST elevation myocardial infarction is still ongoing. Indeed, PPCI results in better patient survival than does fibrinolysis; thus it seems reasonable to argue for a broader application of the mechanical approach. In the meantime, however, it should be realized that the prognosis of myocardial infarction patients strongly depends on the time that has elapsed since the beginning of the coronary occlusion, regardless of the applied reperfusion strategy. The mortality reduction by fibrinolysis as compared to conservative treatment is particularly large if such therapy is initiated within the first 1 or 2 h after symptom onset (Figures 2.3 and 2.4). The additional mortality reduction by PPCI appears to be particularly large if the first balloon inflation is performed within approximately half an hour after a first injection with a fibrinolytic agent would have been possible (Figure 2.6). Hence, all those involved in the care of myocardial infarction patients should be encouraged to optimize prehospital and in-hospital logistic procedures in order to enable treatment in these narrow time windows. Prehospital triage is crucial.

REFERENCES

1. Herrick JB. Clinical features of sudden obstruction of the coronary arteries. J Am Med Assoc 1912; 59: 2015

2. DeWood MA, Spores J, Notske R, et al. Prevalence of total coronary artery occlusion during the early hours of transmural myocardial infarction. N Engl J Med 1980; 303: 897–902

3. Flameng W, Lesaffre E, Vanhaecke J. Determinants of infarct size in non-human primates. Bas Res Cardiol 1990; 85: 392–403

4. Reimer KA, van der Heide RS, Richard VJ. Reperfusion in acute myocardial infarction: effect of timing and modulating factors in experimental models. Am J Cardiol 1993; 72 (Suppl): 13G–21G

5. Reimer KA, Lowe JE, Rasmussen MM, Jennings RB. The wavefront phenomenon of ischemic cell death. 1. Myocardial infarct size versus duration of coronary occlusion in dogs. Circulation 1977; 56: 786–94

6. Dorado DG, Théroux P, Elizaga J, et al. Myocardial infarction in the pig heart model: infarct size and duration of coronary occlusion. Cardiovasc Res 1987; 21: 537–44

7. Schaper W, Binz K, Sass S, Winkler B. Influence of collateral blood flow and of variations in MVO2 on tissue-ATP content in ischemic and infarcted myocardium. J Mol Cell Cardiol 1987; 19: 19–37

8. Hermens WT, Willems GM, Nijssen KM, Simoons ML. Effect of thrombolytic treatment delay on myocardial infarction size [Letter to the editor]. Lancet 1992; 340: 1297

9. Fibrinolytic Therapy Trialists' (FTT) Collaborative Group. Indications for fibrinolytic therapy in suspected acute myocardial infarction: collaborative overview of early mortality and major morbidity results from all randomised trials of more than 1,000 patients. Lancet 1994; 343: 311–22

10. Boersma E, Maas ACP, Deckers JW, Simoons ML. Early thrombolytic treatment in acute myocardial infarction: reappraisal of the golden hour. Lancet 1996; 348: 771–5

11. Grines CL. Should thrombolysis or primary angioplasty be the treatment of choice for acute myocardial infarction? Primary angioplasty – the strategy of choice. N Engl J Med 1996; 335: 1313–16

12. Meijer A, Verheugt FW, Werter CJ, Lie KI, Van der Pol JM, Van Eenige MJ. Aspirin versus coumadin in the prevention of reocclusion and recurrent ischemia after successful thrombolysis: a prospective placebo-controlled angiographic study. Results of the APRI-COT Study. Circulation 1993; 87: 1524–30

13. The GUSTO Angiographic Investigators. The effects of tissue plasminogen activator, streptokinase, or both on coronary-artery patency, ventricular function, and survival after acute myocardial infarction. N Engl J Med 1993; 329: 1615–22

14. Weaver WD, Simes RJ, Betriu A, et al. Comparison of primary coronary angioplasty and intravenous thrombolytic therapy for acute myocardial infarction: a quantitative review. J Am Med Assoc 1997; 278: 2093–8

15. Keeley EC, Boura JA, Grines CL. Primary angioplasty versus intravenous thrombolytic therapy for acute myocardial infarction: a quantitative review of 23 randomised trials. Lancet 2003; 361: 13–20

16. De Luca G, van't Hof AW, de Boer MJ, et al. Time-to-treatment significantly affects the extent of ST-segment resolution and myocardial blush in patients with acute myocardial infarction treated by primary angioplasty. Eur Heart J 2004; 25: 1009–13

17. Brodie BR, Stuckey TD, Wall TC, et al. Importance of time to reperfusion for 30-day and late survival and recovery of left ventricular function after primary angioplasty for acute myocardial infarction. J Am Coll Cardiol 1998; 32: 1312–19

18. Cannon CP, Gibson CM, Lambrew CT, et al. Relationship of symptom-onset-to-balloon time and door-to-balloon time with mortality in patients undergoing angioplasty for acute myocardial infarction. J Am Med Assoc 2000; 283: 2941–7

19. Boersma E, Simes J, Grines C, Westerhout C, on behalf of the PCAT-2 investigators. Does time matter? Individual patient data-based meta-analysis of primary PCI versus fibrinolysis in acute myocardial infarction randomized trials. Data presented at the Annual Scientific Sessions of the American Heart Association, New Orleans, 2004

20. Weaver WD. Time to thrombolytic treatment: factors affecting delay and their influence on outcome. J Am Coll Cardiol 1995; 25 (Suppl): 3S–9S

21. Hasdai D, Behar S, Wallentin L, et al. A prospective survey of the characteristics, treatments and outcomes of patients with acute coronary syndromes in Europe and the Mediterranean basin; the Euro Heart Survey of Acute Coronary Syndromes (Euro Heart Survey ACS). Eur Heart J 2002; 23: 1190–201

22. The European Myocardial Infarction Project Group. Prehospital thrombolytic therapy in patients with suspected acute myocardial infarction. N Engl J Med 1993; 329: 383–9

23. Weaver WD, Cerqueira M, Hallstrom AP, et al., for the Myocardial Infarction Triage and Intervention Project Group. Prehospital-initiated vs hospital-initiated thrombolytic therapy. The Myocardial Infarction Triage and Intervention trial. J Am Med Assoc 1993; 270: 1211–16

24. GREAT Group. Feasibility, safety, and efficacy of domiciliary thrombolysis by general practitioners: Grampian region early anistreplase trial. Br Med J 1992; 305: 548–53

25. The Task Force on the management of acute myocardial infarction of the European Society of Cardiology. Acute myocardial infarction: prehospital and inhospital management. Eur Heart J 1996; 17: 43–63

26. The GUSTO investigators. An international randomized trial comparing four thrombolytic strategies for acute myocardial infarction. N Engl J Med 1993; 329: 673–82

27. White H. Thrombin-specific anticoagulation with bivalirudin versus heparin in patients receiving fibrinolytic therapy for acute myocardial infarction: the HERO-2 randomised trial. Lancet 2001; 358: 1855–63

28. Ferguson JD, Brady WJ, Perron AD, et al. The prehospital 12-lead electrocardiogram: impact on management of the out-of-hospital acute coronary syndrome patient. Am J Emerg Med 2003; 21: 136–42

29. Zijlstra F. Angioplasty vs thrombolysis for acute myocardial infarction: a quantitative overview of the effects of interhospital transportation. Eur Heart J 2003; 24: 21–3

30. McNeill AJ, Cunningham SR, Flannery DJ, et al. A double blind placebo controlled study of early and late administration of recombinant tissue plasminogen activator in acute myocardial infarction. Br Heart J 1989; 61: 316–21

31. Schofer J, Büttner J, Geng G, et al. Prehospital thrombolysis in acute myocardial infarction. Am J Cardiol 1990; 66: 1429–33

32. Barbash GI, Roth A, Hod H, et al. Improved survival but not left ventricular function with early and prehospital treatment with tissue plasminogen activator in acute myocardial infarction. Am J Cardiol 1990; 66: 261–6

33. Castaigne AD, Hervé C, Duval-Moulin AM, et al. Pre-hospital use of APSAC: results of a placebo-controlled study. Am J Cardiol 1989; 64 (Suppl): 30A–3A

34. McAleer B, Ruane B, Burke E, et al. Prehospital thrombolysis in a rural community: short- and long-term survival. Cardiovasc Drugs Ther 1992; 6: 369–72

35. Adams J, Trent R, Rawles J, on behalf of the GREAT Group. Earliest electrocardiographic evidence of myocardial infarction: implications for thrombolytic treatment. Br Med J 1993; 307: 409–13

36. Boersma H, Maas ACP, Grijseels EWM, Deckers JW, Harman JAM, Simoons ML. Benefits and risks of possible prehospital thrombolysis strategies – the role of the electrocardiogram. Cardiologie 1998; 5: 562–8

37. Gore JM, Granger CB, Simoons ML, et al., for the GUSTO-1 investigators. Stroke after thrombolysis: mortality and functional outcomes in the GUSTO-1 trial. Circulation 1995; 92: 2811–18

38. Bouten MJM, Simoons ML, Hartman JAM, Van Miltenburg AJM, Van der Does E, Pool J. Prehospital thrombolysis with alteplase (rt-PA) in acute myocardial infarction. Eur Heart J 1992; 13: 925–31

39. Grijseels EW, Bouten MJ, Lenderink T, et al. Pre-hospital thrombolytic therapy with either alteplase or streptokinase. Practical applications, complications and long-term results in 529 patients. Eur Heart J 1995; 16: 1833–8

40. Boersma E, Maas ACP, Hartman JAM, Ilmer B, Vos J, Simoons ML. 12 year triage and thrombolysis treatment prior to hospitalization for myocardial infarction in the Rotterdam area: outstanding short-term and long-term results [in Dutch with summary in English]. Ned Tijdschr Geneesk 2001; 145: 2029–35

41. The GUSTO-3 investigators. A comparison of reteplase with alteplase for acute myocardial infarction. N Engl J Med 1997; 337: 1118–23

42. The ASSENT-2 investigators. Single-bolus tenecteplase compared with front-loaded alteplase in acute myocardial infarction: the ASSENT-2 double-blind randomised trial. Assessment of the Safety and Efficacy of a New Thrombolytic Investigators. Lancet 1999; 354: 716–22

43. Topol EJ. Reperfusion therapy for acute myocardial infarction with fibrinolytic therapy or combination reduced fibrinolytic therapy and platelet glycoprotein IIb/IIIa inhibition: the GUSTO V randomised trial. Lancet 2001; 357: 1905–14

44. The ASSENT-3 investigators. Efficacy and safety of tenecteplase in combination with enoxaparin, abciximab, or unfractionated heparin: the ASSENT-3 randomised trial in acute myocardial infarction. Lancet 2001; 358: 605–13

45. Lamfers EJP, Hooghoudt TEH, Uppelschoten A, Stolwijk PWJ, Verheugt FWA. Effect of prehospital thrombolysis on aborting acute myocardial infarction. Am J Cardiol 1999; 84: 928–30

46. Zijlstra F, van't Hof AW, Liem AL, Hoorntje JC, Suryapranata H, de Boer MJ. Transferring patients for primary angioplasty: a retrospective analysis of 104 selected high risk patients with acute myocardial infarction. Heart 1997; 78: 333–6

47. Dalby M, Bouzamondo A, Lechat P, Montalescot G. Transfer for primary angioplasty versus immediate thrombolysis in acute myocardial infarction: a meta-analysis. Circulation 2003; 108: 1809–14

48. Straumann E, Yoon S, Naegeli B, et al. Hospital transfer for primary coronary angioplasty in high risk patients with acute myocardial infarction. Heart 1999; 82: 415–19

49. Ernst NMSKJ, De Boer MJ, Van't Hof AWJ, et al. Pre-hospital triage for angiography-guided therapy for acute myocardial infarction. Neth Heart J 2004; 12: 151–6

50. Terkelsen CJ, Lassen JF, Norgaard BL, et al. Reduction of treatment delay in patients with ST-elevation myocardial infarction: impact of pre-hospital diagnosis and direct referral to primary percutanous coronary intervention. Eur Heart J 2005; 26: 770–7

51. Ross AM, Coyne KS, Reiner JS, et al. A randomized trial comparing primary angioplasty with a strategy of short-acting thrombolysis and immediate planned rescue angioplasty in acute myocardial infarction: the PACT trial. PACT investigators. Plasminogen-activator Angioplasty Compatibility Trial. J Am Coll Cardiol 1999; 34: 1954–62

52. Kastrati A, Mehilli J, Schlotterbeck K, et al. Early administration of reteplase plus abciximab vs abciximab alone in patients with acute myocardial infarction referred for percutaneous coronary intervention: a randomized controlled trial. J Am Med Assoc 2004; 291: 947–54

53. Fernandez-Aviles F, Alonso JJ, Castro-Beiras A, et al.; for the GRACIA (Grupo de Analisis de la Cardiopatia Isquemica Aguda) Group. Routine invasive strategy within 24 hours of thrombolysis versus ischaemia-guided conservative approach for acute

myocardial infarction with ST-segment elevation (GRACIA-1): a randomised controlled trial. Lancet 2004; 364: 1045–53

54. Brener SJ, Barr LA, Burchenal JE, et al. Randomized, placebo-controlled trial of platelet glycoprotein IIb/IIIa blockade with primary angioplasty for acute myocardial infarction. ReoPro and Primary PTCA Organization and Randomized Trial (RAPPORT) Investigators. Circulation 1998; 98: 734–41

55. Montalescot G, Barragan P, Wittenberg O, et al.; for the ADMIRAL investigators. Platelet glycoprotein IIb/IIIa inhibition with coronary stenting for acute myocardial infarction. N Engl J Med 2001; 344: 1895–903

56. Zorman S, Zorman D, Noc M. Effects of abciximab pretreatment in patients with acute myocardial infarction undergoing primary angioplasty. Am J Cardiol 2002; 90: 533–6

57. Petronio AS, Rovai D, Musumeci G, et al. Effects of abciximab on microvascular integrity and left ventricular functional recovery in patients with acute infarction treated by primary coronary angioplasty. Eur Heart J 2003; 24: 67–76

58. Stone GW, Grines CL, Cox DA, et al.; for the CADILLAC investigators. Comparison of angioplasty with stenting, with or without abciximab, in acute myocardial infarction. N Engl J Med 2002; 346: 957–66

59. Antoniucci D, Rodriguez A, Hempel A, et al. A randomized trial comparing primary infarct artery stenting with or without abciximab in acute myocardial infarction. J Am Coll Cardiol 2003; 42: 1879–85

60. Kong DF, Califf RM, Miller DP, et al. Clinical outcomes of therapeutic agents that block the platelet glycoprotein IIb/IIIa integrin in ischemic heart disease. Circulation 1998; 98: 2829–35

61. Van't Hof AW, Ernst N, de Boer MJ, et al.; for the On-TIME study group. Facilitation of primary coronary angioplasty by early start of a glycoprotein 2b/3a inhibitor: results of the ongoing tirofiban in myocardial infarction evaluation (On-TIME) trial. Eur Heart J 2004; 25: 837–46

62. Montalescot G, Borentain M, Payot L, Collet JP, Thomas D. Early vs late administration of glycoprotein IIb/IIIa inhibitors in primary percutaneous coronary intervention of acute ST-segment elevation myocardial infarction: a meta-analysis. J Am Med Assoc 2004; 292: 362–6

3

General principles of fibrinolytic therapy in acute myocardial infarction

Robert G Wilcox

INTRODUCTION

Functional or mechanical impairment of endothelial integrity may lead stealthily to atherosclerotic plaque formation and acute episodes of vasospasm or localized intravascular thrombosis. In the coronary circulation the clinical consequences might be silent or symptomatic episodes of myocardial ischemia, sometimes progressing over the years to an ischemic cardiomyopathy or, in the presence of a critical flow limiting thrombus, to more profound ischemic events such as unstable angina or myocardial necrosis if the occlusion is not relieved. The degree and consequences of myocardial necrosis (infarction) will depend on the vessel affected, the proximal site, the extent and duration of the occlusion, the extent of other vessel disease and the quality of collateral coronary flow.

In patients with the clinical event of acute myocardial infarction, coronary artery thrombosis was proposed as the underlying pathological cause as early as 1912 by Herrick, but for decades thereafter it was regarded as an epiphenomenon or postmortem artefact.[1] However, the demonstration of fresh occlusive thrombi at postmortem and during acute angiography in preparation for coronary artery bypass surgery eventually led to the acceptance that, in the majority of patients with acute myocardial infarction, the cause is occlusion by fresh platelet-rich thrombus in the vicinity of an eroded or fissured atherosclerotic plaque. Angiography showed that the process may be dynamic, with spontaneous fibrinolysis and restoration of some coronary flow followed by reocclusion occurring over several hours, such that by 24 h as many as 50% of presumed originally occluded vessels may be patent, albeit leaving irreversible ischemic damage to myocardial cells.[2-5] Animal models of coronary occlusion revealed not only the time dependency of the histopathological extent of such ischemic necrosis, but also a peri-infarct zone of muscle potentially viable if reperfusion was re-established and the effects of reperfusion injury minimal.[6-8]

These experimental, pathological and clinical studies of the acute occlusive thrombotic cause of most instances of myocardial infarction, and the potential for damage limitation, coincided with a reawakened interest in the thrombolytic properties of streptokinase and other plasminogen activators, and a surge in understanding of the central role of platelets in acute arterial thrombus formation. Chemical dissolution of an occluding thrombus was soon shown to be feasible and relatively safe when administered by a peripheral vein rather than directly into the infarct-related coronary artery, and resulted in a significant reduction in both short- and long-term mortality. Effective proactive rather than reactive treatment of acute myocardial infarction had arrived.

CLINICAL OPPORTUNITIES

Acute total or sub-total occlusion of a coronary artery usually causes severe chest pain, sweating, hemodynamic instability and the threat of fatal dysrhythmias. The acute episode is most often accompanied by ECG changes of ST elevation over the area of threatened myocardium, or bundle branch block (usually left bundle). In sub-total or transient occlusion intermittent ST depression or T-wave inversion may occur. In this acute phase the patient is at high risk: some 30% die before admission to hospital and another 15% or more in hospital, such that by 1 month 40–50% of patients will have died. Of those who survive, a considerable proportion will be significantly disabled with reduced effort tolerance depending upon the extent of left ventricular damage and the quality of residual function. The risk of re-infarction in the next year varies considerably from ≤5% to ≥40% depending on age and other co-morbidities, the extent of residual coronary artery disease and especially on the quantity and quality of residual left ventricular function.[9]

These clinicopathological associations and the opportunity for damage limitation and improved prognosis, by restoration of coronary artery patency and myocardial perfusion, make the assessment, protection (by defibrillator availability) and proactive treatment of a patient with acute myocardial infarction a medical emergency. The early re-establishment of infarct-related coronary artery patency is crucial. In one study patients treated with thrombolytic therapy who had early and sustained restoration of patency had an in-hospital mortality of ≤5%, those with initial patency who re-occluded 10% and those who failed to re-open at all a mortality of 17%.[10] In the clinical context of an evolving acute myocardial infarction, 'time costs muscle – and muscle buys time'.

RESTORING VESSEL PATENCY

There are currently two major options for restoring timely patency of an occluded coronary artery: immediate coronary angiography with a view to angioplasty and stent (or in some instances coronary artery bypass surgery); or chemical thrombolysis. For the majority of patients worldwide chemical thrombolysis will be the only available option.

Thrombolytic drugs, of which the bacterially derived streptokinase is the archetype, work by enhancing the conversion of naturally occurring plasminogen within the circulation to the protease enzyme plasmin: they are not direct acting lytics of a thrombus, it is the generated plasmin that digests fibrinogen and fibrin which, together with platelets, are the structural proteins of occlusive thrombi (Figure 3.1). Rather than circulating plasminogen, that bound within an occluding thrombus is obviously a more attractive target for a thrombolytic drug, for this has the potential advantage of generating local clot-bound plasmin rather than a more systemic state of hyperplasminemia and the associated increased risk of bleeding. Whereas streptokinase activates circulating plasminogen but has poor penetrance into thrombi, the next generation of bioengineered derivatives of naturally occurring tissue plasminogen activator (t-PA) have enhanced plasminogen activation in the presence of clot-bound thrombin with the potential for more concentrated local rather than systemic plasmin generation and activity. Such thrombolytics are termed 'clot specific', although they do cause some systemic plasminogen conversion and do not differentiate between clots in different vascular territories, a weakness which in part may be responsible for their most dangerous unwanted effect of intracerebral hemorrhage.

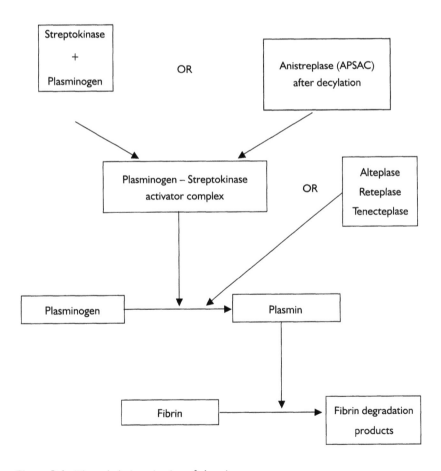

Figure 3.1 Thrombolytic activation of plasminogen.

Of course there are limitations to the effectiveness of thrombolytic therapy. For instance, a ruptured plaque within the infarct-related coronary artery may mechanically prevent prograde penetration of systemically formed plasmin or of an intravenously administered thrombolytic drug, or an extensive column of thrombus may spread not only distally from the site of the initial lesion, but also proximally, perhaps impairing perfusion of branching collateral vessels. Such an extensive 'clot burden' may prove an unassailable obstacle to permeation of plasmin or a thrombolytic drug. There is some possibility too that the constituents of an occlusive thrombus may vary with extent and time, making it less susceptible to digestion by plasmin; hence the urgency to initiate thrombolytic treatment and the search for more effective alternative thrombolytic drugs and anti-thrombotic co-treatments.

CLINICAL TRIALS OF THROMBOLYSIS

General comments

Streptokinase was first used in acute myocardial infarction (AMI) in 1958 and was followed by a number of rather small inconclusive studies of varying dose schedules and reported bleeding risks; then interest waned.[11] Following the pathological and acute angiographic reports described above and two short reports of an experience of intracoronary streptokinase,[12,13] several large controlled phase III trials of streptokinase, streptokinase–plasminogen complex and recombinant tissue plasminogen activator were reported in the late 1980s.[14–17] All showed a reduction in early (28–35 days) mortality irrespective of thrombolytic type and emphasized the declining efficacy when thrombolysis was initiated late after symptom onset. In addition, the increased risk of bleeding, especially of intracerebral bleeds, and the allergic-hypotensive potential of streptokinase was documented.

From these and other smaller controlled trials, a meta-analysis published in 1994 provided an overall assessment of the benefits and risks from thrombolytic therapy and indicated those patient features which might be associated with no benefit or even harm (Tables 3.1 and 3.2).[18] Overall the survival benefit is modest, an extra two or three lives saved per 100 patients treated, albeit with an increased risk of total stroke of about 0.4%. These controlled trials were carried out at a time when image acquisition for stroke was not universal and the figures are probably underestimates. The benefit, however, is sustained over many years.[19]

Table 3.1 Overview of risk/benefit ratio from thrombolysis in acute myocardial infarction

	Control (%)	Fibrinolytic (%)
Mortality 35 days	11.5	9.6
Stroke 35 days*	0.8	1.2
Major bleeds*	0.4	1.1

*Majority in hospital

Adapted from the Fibrinolytic Therapy Trialists' Collaborative Group (1994) (reference 18)

Adding antiplatelet therapy

Aspirin

Aspirin inhibits the platelet enzyme cyclo-oxygenase, thereby inhibiting the production of thromboxane A_2 from arachidonic acid. This inhibition reduces the expression of platelet surface glycoprotein IIb/IIIa receptors, which are instrumental in platelet–fibrinogen–platelet bonding that results in platelet aggregation. One substantial trial, ISIS-2, compared the efficacy of streptokinase, aspirin, both or neither in 17 187 patients.[15] The 35-day cardiovascular mortality according to treatment was 13.2% for placebo, 10.4% for streptokinase, 10.7% for aspirin and 8.0% for combined aspirin plus streptokinase, a 5% absolute reduction in cardio-vascular death with combined therapy, i.e. a saving of five lives per 100 patients treated. This pivotal trial led to aspirin being recommended as initial co-treatment irrespective of which thrombolytic was used.

Clopidogrel

Clopidogrel, a derivative of ticlopidine, is an oral pro-drug whose active metabolism irreversibly inhibits $P2Y_{12}$, a platelet surface receptor for the agonist adenosine diphosphate. The potential additive effect of clopidogrel in patients thrombolysed

Table 3.2 Benefit from thrombolysis according to baseline demographic features

Group	Control group death (%)	Treatment benefit/ 1000 patients
Men	10.1	19
Women	16.0	18
Age (years)		
< 55	4.6	11
55–64	8.9	18
65–74	16.1	27
> 75	25.3	10
Prior MI		
yes	14.1	16
no	10.9	20
Diabetes		
yes	17.3	37
no	10.2	15
ECG		
bundle branch block	23.6	49
anterior ST raised	16.9	37
inferior ST raised	8.4	8
ST depression	13.8	-14
other abnormal	5.8	6
normal	2.3	-7

Adapted from the Fibrinolytic Therapy Trialists' Collaborative Group (1994) (reference 18)

and taking aspirin for AMI was recently reported in two trials. The first was an early culprit artery patency study which showed an absolute 6.7% reduction in the rates of a composite endpoint, comprising occlusion of the infarct-related artery on angiography or death or recurrent myocardial infarction, from 21.7% to 15.0%.[20] The preliminary results of a trial to evaluate the potential survival benefit of this regimen (the COMMIT/CCS-2 trial) was recently reported at the 2005 meeting of the American College of Cardiology (submitted for publication). By hospital discharge total mortality was reduced from 8.1% to 7.7% ($2p = 0.03$) and death/reinfarctions/stroke from 10.1% to 9.3% ($2p = 0.002$). Whether these results will impact on the pharmacological treatment of patients with AMI awaits further critical analysis.

Improving treatment schedules

The next major step in thrombolytic therapy was the GUSTO-1 trial which compared streptokinase (with subcutaneous or intravenous heparin) and a newly described 90-min bolus-infusion 'accelerated' schedule of alteplase with intravenous heparin, and a combination arm of reduced-dose streptokinase plus alteplase; all treatment groups included aspirin.[21,22] The 30-day overall mortality was a significant 1% ($\pm 0.6\%$) lower with the alteplase schedule, thus giving the potential for a further small reduction in overall mortality. Unfortunately the cost differential between streptokinase and alteplase prevented its widespread adoption as the preferred lytic in many countries.

The search for simpler treatment schedules – bolus thrombolytics

Tissue plasminogen activator (t-PA) is produced by the vascular endothelium and is neutralized by plasminogen activator inhibitors. Alteplase (rt-PA) is the recombinant tissue plasminogen activator that is produced by recombinant DNA technology. Several derivatives of rt-PA have been synthesized and three of them (reteplase, lanoteplase and tenecteplase) have been compared with alteplase in phase III outcome studies. These derivatives vary minimally (tenecteplase) or substantially (reteplase) from the parent molecule, but the property they share in common and which has been exploited therapeutically is a longer half-life permitting bolus rather than infusion administration (Figure 3.2). Tenecteplase, in addition, has some resistance to tissue plasminogen activator inhibitors. Both reteplase and lanoteplase lack the finger domain of the parent molecule and thus have lower affinities for fibrin than alteplase, whereas tenecteplase has more. Antigenicity has not been a problem with any of these new molecules.

The possibility of bolus administration of a thrombolytic drug increases the possibility of more rapid treatment after patient assessment in the receiving room, and the real opportunities for very early treatment in the community, where most heart attacks occur.

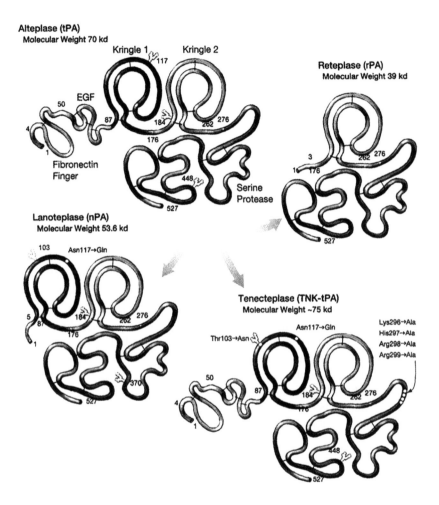

Figure 3.2 Structure of various thrombolytic agents. The structure–function relationships for the various domains are as follows: kringle 1, receptor binding (liver); kringle 2, fibrin binding (low affinity); fibronectin finger, fibrin binding (high affinity); epidermal growth factor, hepatic clearance; serine protease, catalytic activity and plasminogen activator inhibitor 1 binding; glycosylation sites, clearance via hepatic endothelial cells.

Reproduced with permission from Llevadot J, Giugliano RP, Antman EM: J Am Med Assoc 2001; 286: 442–9. Copyrighted (2001), American Medical Association.

Reteplase (rPA)

The half-life of this bioengineered tPA led to the investigation of double-bolus intravenous injections separated by 30 min. After two coronary artery patency studies against 'original' 3-h alteplase infusion and 'accelerated' 90-min alteplase (RAPID 1 and 2), a double-bolus 10 MU schedule, separated by 30 min, was chosen for comparison with streptokinase in patients with acute myocardial infarction (INJECT study).[23] This was a pivotal trial in cardiovascular medicine, for it introduced the concept of equivalence of efficacy between two drugs rather than attempting to assert superiority. Equivalence has clinical as well as statistical boundaries and allows the testing of a new drug in a clinical situation where a placebo comparator would not be ethical. In the event that equivalence is proven, then in order to be preferred against a proven and long-established comparator, the new drug must confer other advantages, such as ease of administration, lower cost or fewer unwanted effects.

In the INJECT trial of 6010 patients randomized within 12 h of symptom onset of AMI, the 35-day mortality rates were 9.0% for reteplase and 9.5% for streptokinase; both the predefined clinical and statistical definitions of equivalence were satisfied. As with other tissue plasminogen activators, there was a higher total stroke rate for reteplase (1.23% vs. 1.00%) and comparable serious bleeds (0.7% reteplase vs. 1.0% streptokinase).

The same reteplase schedule was then compared with the GUSTO-1 accelerated alteplase schedule in the GUSTO-3 trial of 15 059 patients, but because of the 90-min patency superiority of reteplase seen in RAPID 2 (59.9% vs. 45.2%) a more ambitious survival superiority for reteplase was sought.[24] Mortality at 30 days (7.5% vs. 7.2%, respectively) and at 1 year (11.2% vs. 11.1%, respectively) was comparable, as were the overall rates of total stroke and other major bleeding complications. Superiority, therefore, was not proven.

Despite the failure to assert superiority over accelerated alteplase, the results of INJECT and GUSTO-3 provided the cardiologist with the first bolus tissue plasminogen activator schedule.

Lanoteplase (n-PA)

After similar modest-sized dose-finding coronary artery patency studies, a single dose of 120 kU/kg dose of lanoteplase (n-PA) was compared with accelerated alteplase in a 15 078 patient equivalence trial, IN-TIME II.[25] The 30-day mortality rates (6.75% lanoteplase vs. 6.61% alteplase) satisfied the equivalence definition of the trial and this persisted at the 6-month follow-up (8.7% vs. 8.8%, respectively). Unexpectedly, the rate of intracerebral hemorrhage (ICH) for lanoteplase was significantly higher than for alteplase (1.12% vs. 0.64%, $p = 0.004$), although this was the lowest ICH rate ever recorded for any alteplase trial with strict imaging acquisition and verification. There was also an increased incidence of minor bleeds with lanoteplase (19.7% vs. 14.8%, $p < 0.0001$). Whatever the cause of the increased bleeding complications – the dose of lanoteplase, the heparin schedule, the age composition of the patient group or the lower fibrin specificity of lanoteplase – it was decided not to pursue the drug for therapeutic use. However, the lessons learnt from the follow-on smaller IN-TIME IIb lower heparin schedule study led to important changes for adjunctive heparin dosage and the recommendation for earlier assessment of the activated partial thromboplastin time by the ACC/AHA Guidelines Committee.

Tenecteplase (TNK-tPA)

In contrast to the modest-sized phase II dose-finding studies carried out with reteplase and lanoteplase, tenecteplase underwent extensive phase II patency and safety studies in the TIMI-IOB (837 patients) and ASSENT-I (3325 patients) trials. An ICH rate of 0.62% was seen with the 40-mg dose combined with the now recommended lower heparin schedule.

The ASSENT-2 trial therefore compared a single bolus of tenecteplase 30–50 mg (depending on body weight) with accelerated alteplase in a 16 949 patient AMI trial.[26] Equivalent mortality rates were observed at 30 days (6.18% vs. 6.15%) which persisted at 1 year. ICH rates, too, were comparable (0.93% tenecteplase vs. 0.94% alteplase), although these were higher than hoped for from the phase II safety data.

Summary of bolus thrombolytic therapy

These three trials established equivalent efficacy in terms of total mortality or the clinical composite of death plus non-fatal disabling stroke of gold standard accelerated alteplase and bolus therapy. They also ushered in new recommendations regarding heparin dosing and the timing of APTT checks on its anticoagulant activity. Although lanoteplase has been abandoned, both reteplase and tenecteplase are now available as bolus therapies (double or single bolus, respectively) and have virtually replaced the more complex 90-min accelerated alteplase schedule. They are also being assessed (and promoted) as out-of-hospital thrombolytic treatments for patients in the very early throes of acute myocardial infarction where the greatest gains in mortality reduction (and possibly infarct abortion) are expected.

VESSEL PATENCY AND MICROVASCULAR PERFUSION

The goal of thrombolytic therapy is to achieve a patent infarct-related artery in the shortest possible time following symptom onset, with the lowest incidence of side-effects. In GUSTO-1 a substantial angiographic sub-study was carried out which confirmed the relationship between vessel patency and 30-day mortality (Figure 3.3) However, this was achieved in only 54% of patients with the most effective accelerated alteplase schedule.[27] Furthermore, early reocclusion occurs in 5–25% of treated patients depending on the thrombolytic and adjunctive therapies used.[27,28] Thus, the establishment and maintenance of early patency became the 'holy grail' of thrombolytic therapy, indeed of any reperfusion therapy. Despite the encouraging phase II superior early patency data obtained with the third-generation bolus thrombolytics (reteplase, lanoteplase and tenecteplase) described earlier, none have reduced mortality beyond that already achieved with accelerated alteplase. However, their ease of administration will ensure a role in the very early prehospital treatment area, a therapeutic opportunity largely ignored despite some optimistic earlier studies and local pockets of enthusiasm.[29]

Part of the explanation for this discrepancy between achieved patency and survival came from studies in which myocardial perfusion was assessed in addition

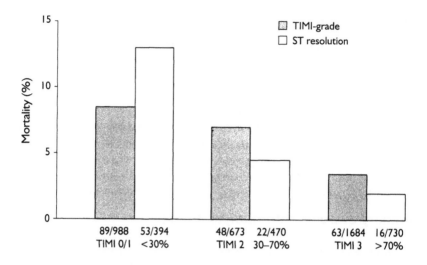

Figure 3.3 The 90-min TIMI patency grade and 30-day mortality following thrombolysis for acute myocardial infarction.
From the GUSTO Angiographic Investigators (1993) (reference 27).

to epicardial vessel patency.[30,31] Between 25 and 50% of patients may have suboptimal perfusion despite optimal patency (the so-called no reflow phenomenon).[32] This has complex causes which include microvascular emboli, microvascular edema and the release of leukocyte cytokines.[33] In the search for speedier, more sustained vessel patency and improved microvascular perfusion, attention therefore shifted towards more powerful concomitant anti-thrombin and anti-platelet therapies. Thus large phase II/III trials with enoxaparin, a low molecular weight heparin (ASSENT III), abciximab, a platelet glycoprotein IIb/IIIa receptor blocker (ASSENT III, GUSTO V), and hirudin, a direct acting anti-thrombin (HERO-2) have all been conducted and will be described in detail in subsequent chapters. Suffice it here to say that none reduced the incidence of total mortality beyond that of established comparator thrombolytic schedules, nor of hemorrhagic stroke, but there were encouraging reductions of recurrent in-hospital ischemic events, the clinical significance of which will emerge only with longer follow-up data.

PROBLEMS WITH THROMBOLYTICS

Stroke

The excess stroke risk that accompanies thrombolytic use is due to intracerebral hemorrhage, usually occurring within the first 24 h, and results in death in about 60% of affected patients, thereby contributing significantly to the overall mortality in treated patients and limiting the full potential of thrombolytic therapy. Hopes that hemorrhagic stroke risk would be reduced by the use of 'clot-specific' tissue plasminogen activator derivatives were dashed by several subsequent 'head to head' comparator trials described above. In general, hemorrhagic stroke risk after streptokinase is ≤0.5% and after a tissue plasminogen activator 0.5–1.0%. The complicity of concomitant antithrombotic therapy with heparin in these events is an on-going debate.[34] From the demographic and outcome data available from the thrombolytic trials, Simoons and colleagues published a model from which it may be possible to predict the likely risk of intracerebral hemorrhage.[35] Although this has not been tested prospectively, some clinicians refer to it when choosing between streptokinase and tissue plasminogen activators, or avoiding thrombolysis altogether, for instance in a light-weight elderly woman with a 'small' inferior infarction.

Bleeding

Giving a thrombolytic drug, an anti-platelet and an anti-thrombin obviously increases the bleeding risk (Table 3.1), especially if the APPT is allowed to drift too high. Bleeds may occur spontaneously anywhere, but are more likely in the presence of covert bleeding areas (bowel, bladder) and especially at the sites of vascular puncture. The majority, however, are minor ecchymoses; the most serious, endangering life or neurological function, are intracranial bleeds, as described earlier.

Anaphylaxis

This occurs rarely in patients treated with a tissue plasminogen activator, but in ≤2% of patients given streptokinase. It is usually mild but can be life threatening in the event of a severe acute autoimmune-type response. Hypotension may occur in ≤10% of streptokinase-treated patients and can usually be treated with temporary cessation of the infusion (or switch to a tissue plasminogen activator if available), fluid replacement and atropine if associated with bradycardia. Antibodies to streptokinase may last many years and theoretically could negate the benefit of further exposure, or provoke an anaphylactic reaction.[36] In ideal circumstances, streptokinase should be a 'once-in-a-lifetime' drug.[37]

Failed thrombolysis and 'rescue'

It may be difficult to assert whether or not thrombolysis has been successful. If the patient remains in pain and the ECG shows persistent ST segment elevation, then either patency or reperfusion has not been achieved. Schröder and colleagues promoted the principle of ST segment elevation resolution, i.e. return to the isoelectric line, arbitrarily divided into no resolution, ≤30% resolution and ≥70% resolution.[38] This procedure was tested prospectively and compared with angiographic evidence of both patency (and later with perfusion too) and subsequently mortality (Figure 3.4).[32,39] Despite the excellent correlation, there remains uncertainty about which strategy to adopt – treat symptomatically with analgesia, anti-ischemic and anti-coagulant therapy, or a repeat trial of thrombolysis,

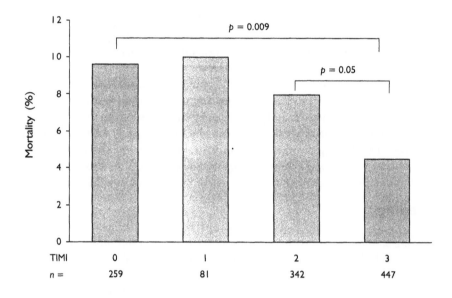

Figure 3.4 'Open artery' versus 'relief of ischemia'. TIMI 0, 1, 2, 3 is assessment of coronary patency, and < 30%, 30–70%, > 70% assessment of ST segment resolution. From Schröder *et al*. (1995) (reference 39).

or proceed to coronary angiography with a view to intervention. Limited controlled and uncontrolled data suggested that the latter policy is excellent if the intervention is successful, but disastrous if not![40]

Recently the results of the REACT trial were presented at the 2004 American Heart Association meeting (submitted for publication). In that trial, patients treated with thrombolysis for AMI and whose ECG failed to show > 50% ST segment resolution at 90 min from start of treatment, were randomly allocated to continue with supportive medical treatment, to further lytic treatment using a tissue plasminogen activator (i.e. not a second dose of streptokinase), or to angiography with a view to percutaneous coronary intervention/coronary artery bypass graft (PCI/CABG). By 6 months there was a significant reduction in the composite endpoint of all-cause mortality/re-myocardial infarction/severe heart failure/stroke from 30% in the two non-interventional arms to 15% in the invasive arm ($p = 0.003$). The reduction in total mortality from 12% to 6% was not significant.

These new findings on rescue angioplasty when reviewed in the context of existing data could pose major logistic problems in care provision.

After thrombolysis, then what?

All patients recovering from an acute myocardial infarction should be actively considered for prophylactic treatment with a number of proven therapies: aspirin, an angiotensin converting enzyme (ACE) inhibitor, β-blocker, a statin and, in those with early left ventricular dysfunction and pulmonary edema, eplerenone, an aldos-terone antagonist lacking the estrogenic effects of spironolactone.[41] The usefulness of long-term anti-inflammatory therapy is not yet proven. The role of routine early exercise testing in the asymptomatic patient to 'expose residual ischemia' remains controversial, but there is some evidence of benefit provided a coronary intervention can be offered.[42,43]

Routine angiography after thrombolysis

If successful, thrombolytic therapy will result in dissolution of the occluding fresh thrombus, albeit in only 50–60% of patients. The pre-existing atherosclerotic plaque remains unscathed and so may promote reocclusion until all the 'inflammatory' activity has resolved, or prevent adequate prograde flow such that recurrent myocardial ischemia may occur.

In the late 1980s, a series of randomized trials (e.g. TAMI, ECSG, TIMI 2A) compared routine with 'as necessary' intervention in the asymptomatic survivors of AMI and failed to show benefit. In the new era of balloon-mounted and coated stents, this issue has been re-addressed in the GRACIA trial.[44] In this trial 500 thrombolysed patients were randomized to angiography within 24 h or as deemed clinically necessary. The primary endpoint of death/reinfarctions/revascularization by 1 year was reduced from 21% to 9% by early intervention ($p = 0.0008$). However, this result excluded the protocol-mandated interventions in the 'aggressively' treated group of patients. If these procedures are added, then early intervention increases the composite endpoint from 21% to 96% ($p < 0.0001$), the exact opposite of what the GRACIA investigators claimed. Perhaps waiting to intervene until clinically necessary as opposed to routinely proceeding to angiography should prevail on current evidence?

PATIENT SELECTION FOR THROMBOLYTIC THERAPY

The Fibrinolytic Therapy Trialists (FTT) overview suggested that, of those patients deemed initially eligible for thrombolysis, i.e. not considered to have a significant bleeding risk, the groups not likely to benefit were those whose initial electro-cardiogram was either normal, equivocal, or showed ECG ST segment depression rather than elevation (Tables 3.1 and 3.2). Even in the elderly, some overall benefit was retained; although in the context of general use rather than in the context of a clinical trial setting, this assertion has been challenged.[45]

In general, in the absence of an experienced immediately available primary angioplasty service, thrombolysis should be considered for every patient presenting within 12 h of onset of chest pain considered to be due to myocardial ischemia and whose ECG shows either ST elevation or bundle branch block (thought to be new, but often difficult to be certain in practice). Beyond 12 h there may be little myocardium left to 'salvage', but in the presence of continuing pain and ST elevation and the uncertainty of the timing of infarction, offering thrombolytic treatment would seem reasonable.

It is not reasonable, however, to withhold thrombolysis in a patient with proliferative diabetic retinopathy or after cardiopulmonary resuscitation, but in the presence of hypotension an alternative to streptokinase is to be preferred lest further blood pressure lowering occurs. In view of the uncertain consequences of strepto-kinase antibodies in a previously treated patient, it is probably prudent to avoid re-exposure at all if alternative drugs are available. Even if re-administered within 48 h before significant antibodies appear, its therapeutic use may be reduced by virtue of low plasma plasminogen which was 'consumed' by the earlier dose.

Prehospital thrombolysis, on-site thrombolysis, or transfer to an interventional center

The maximum potential from a thrombolytic strategy is likely only to be realized if treatment could be started as soon as possible after symptom onset (Figure 3.5).[46] This would necessitate a significant reduction in the patient delay to calling for medical assistance, a rapid medical response and the initiation of treatment out of hospital, either by paramedic personnel or attending primary care physicians. The availability now of bolus rather than intravenous infusion thrombolytic schedules makes prehospital thrombolysis an urgent priority for widespread implementation.

A meta-analysis of all available trials comparing on-site thrombolysis with primary PCI favored intervention for a reduction in all-cause early mortality (7% vs.

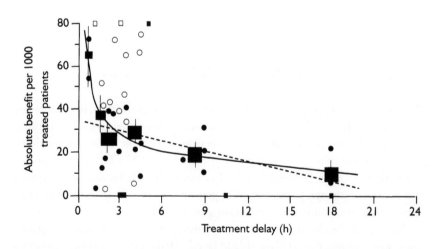

Figure 3.5 Relationship between treatment delay and absolute benefit per 1000 treated patients.
Symbols represent the results of individual trials entered in the analysis.
Reproduced with permission from the Lancet (1996) (reference 46).

Table 3.3 Transfer for primary percutaneous coronary intervention (PCI) versus thrombo-lysis on site. (MAARSTRICHT, PRAGUE 1, AIR-PAMI, CAPTIM*, DANAMI-2, PRAGUE 2)

% events	PCI (n = 1887)	Thrombolysis (n = 1963)
Death, reinfarctions, stroke	7.8	13.4
death	6.3	7.7 (p = 0.086)
reinfarctions	1.5	5.0 (p < 0.001)
stroke	0.6	1.8 (p = 0.015)

*CAPTIM, prehospital lysis
From Dalby et al. (reference 48)

9%), non-fatal re-myocardial infarction (3% vs. 7%) and intracerebral hemorrhage (0.5% vs.1%).[47] Although the conclusion is not as robust for those patients who were thrombolysed with t-PA rather than streptokinase, the results were regarded as sufficiently persuasive to suggest trials of on-site thrombolysis versus transport from the receiving hospital to a center capable of performing primary PCI. Several such studies have been concluded and despite transport distances sometimes exceeding 100 km, overviews suggest benefit (Table 3.3).[48]

Individual trials invite criticism: for instance, patient selection for transport, streptokinase as a comparator therapy, exclusion of procedural infarcts from the combined endpoint and over-enthusiastic extrapolation of the results to suggest transfer for all patients with acute infarction. Transfer incurs an inevitable delay before reperfusion therapy can begin: precious time during which myocytes are succumbing to ischemia. One critical analysis of this 'delay to balloon' reperfusion has suggested that the longer the time differential between thrombolysis and PCI the smaller the apparent benefit from PCI, such that by 60 min there is no survival benefit at all.[49] This observation accords with findings from the PRAGUE 2 and CAPTIM trials.[50,51] In PRAGUE 2, an on-site versus transfer trial, those patients who received thrombolytic therapy within 3 h of symptom onset (with streptokinase in this trial) had the same 30-day mortality as those randomized to transfer for PCI within the same time period (7.4% vs. 7.3%, respectively).

The CAPTIM trial is the only trial to date where out-of-hospital thrombolysis has been compared with transport to a PCI center. In this French trial of 840 patients, not only did prehospital thrombolysed patients have a similar 30-day mortality (3.4%) to those transported for PCI (4.3%), but those treated within 2 h of symptom onset did better (2.2% vs. 5.8%, p = 0.058).

The logistics of preferential transport to an interventional center or of transfer from a non-interventional center in order to offer primary PCI as opposed to thrombolysis anywhere are formidable, but from the above examples these can be overcome. However, out-of-hospital thrombolysis with modern bolus lytics and ancillary anticoagulants (aspirin, subcutaneous low molecular weight heparin and possibly clopidogrel) might still be a viable and sensible option.

CLINICAL GUIDELINES AND TREATMENT SCHEDULES

For common clinical guidelines and contraindications see Table 3.4, but also review the information inserts for a particular product.[52] Of the contraindications listed some may be of lesser risk than others and for some clear evidence lacking, so clinical judgement will often be needed. A history of hypertension but with preliminary good control and 'normal' value on admission or a previously normotensive patient with elevated levels on admission, whether or not reduced by medical therapy, remain difficult judgement issues. In the absence of easily available alternative therapy with percutaneous transluminal coronary angioplasty (PTCA), then streptokinase (if previously not given) might be the lytic of choice, but even its information insert gives ambiguous advice. If clinical judgement suggests that the intracerebral bleeding risk is higher than the expected benefit, then the lytic should be withheld.

Table 3.4 Thrombolysis in acute myocardial infarct: indications and contraindications

Indications

Clinical presentation consistent with myocardial infarction within the previous 12 h and at least one of:
1 mm ST elevation in two or more contiguous limb leads
2 mm ST elevation in two or more contiguous limb leads
New (presumed or known) left bundle branch block
Consider in patients presenting 12–24 h if chest pain and ST elevation are persisting

Absolute contraindications*

Hemorrhage stroke or stroke of unknown origin at any time
Ischemic stroke in preceding 6 months
Central nervous system damage or neoplasms
Recent major trauma/surgery/head injury within preceding 3 weeks
Gastrointestinal bleeding within the last month
Known bleeding disorder
Aortic dissection

Relative contraindications*

Transient ischemic attack in preceding 6 months
Oral anticoagulant therapy
Pregnancy or within 1 week postpartum
Non-compressible vascular punctures
Traumatic resuscitation
Refractory hypertension (systolic blood pressure > 180 mmHg)
Advanced liver disease
Infective endocarditis
Active peptic ulcer

*From the Task Force on the Management of AMI of the European Society of Cardiology (2003) (reference 52)

Table 3.5 Fibrinolytic regimens for acute myocardial infarction*

Fibrinolytic	Initial treatment	Antithrombin	Contraindications
Streptokinase	1.5 million units in 100 ml 5% dextrose or 0.9% saline over 30–60 min	None or i.v. heparin for 24–48 h	Prior SK or anistreplase
Alteplase	15 mg i.v. bolus 0.75 mg/kg over 30 min i.v. 0.5 mg/kg over 60 min i.v. Total dose ≤ 100 mg	i.v. heparin for 24–48 h	
Reteplase	10 U + 10 U i.v. bolus given 30 min apart	i.v. heparin for 24–48 h	
Tenecteplase	single i.v. bolus of 30 mg if < 60 kg 35 mg if 60 to < 70 kg 40 mg if 70 to < 80 kg 45 mg if 80 to < 90 kg 50 mg if ≥ 90 kg	i.v. heparin for 24–48 h	

*From the Task Force on the Management of AMI of the European Society of Cardiology (2003) (reference 52)

Current fibrinolytic schedules are given in Table 3.5; all include co-treatment with oral aspirin.[52] Adjunctive treatment with heparin has never been proven to reduce mortality irrespective of the fibrinolytic drug used. It is recommended especially in conjunction with a tissue plasminogen activator (alteplase, reteplase, tenecteplase) purely on the basis of phase II coronary artery patency trials. The optimum dose, duration and anticoagulant intensity are not known, but recent advice would be to monitor APPT early, to keep within 55–70 seconds and to employ weight adjustment normograms.[34] These regimens may change according to local interpretation of trials incorporating low molecular weight heparin, direct acting anti-thrombins, or platelet glycoprotein IIb/IIIa inhibitors.

CONCLUDING COMMENTS

Thrombolytic therapy with concomitant aspirin (and possibly heparin) has reduced the risk of death in eligible patients by about 40%. There are problems concerning the time delay between symptom onset and treatment prescription which can only be resolved by out-of-hospital therapy. The cheapest drug, streptokinase, does have antigenic potential and is not ideally suitable for prehospital treatment as an infusion, but the newer bolus lytics are (reteplase and tenecteplase). Whereas aspirin co-treatment seems essential, other adjunctive therapies remain to be proven and will be discussed in following chapters. The issue of risk, especially from intracranial hemorrhage, undoubtedly has a negative impact on prescribing behavior in some countries more than others, but what remains inexplicable is the underuse of lytics in apparently lytic-eligible patients.[53,54] Whereas 50% or more of patients with acute myocardial infarction appear eligible for thrombolysis, up to a quarter of them do not receive it or any other reperfusion therapy, and they have a higher mortality.[55] Finally, a significant proportion of patients are considered ineligible for thrombolysis and without the option of coronary angioplasty or timely coronary artery bypass surgery these patients have long been known to have a mortality several-fold higher than that of thrombolyzed patients.[56,57] To date there have been few attempts to test alternative strategies in this heterogeneous very high-risk group of patients. One trial using the glycoprotein IIb/IIIa inhibitor tirofiban was neutral. Preliminary data from the COMMIT/CCS-2 trial mentioned earlier suggests slight benefit from clopidogrel in non-reperfused patients, but further data analysis is awaited.

REFERENCES

1. Herrick JB. Clinical features of sudden obstruction of the coronary arteries. J Am Med Assoc 1912; 59: 2015–20

2. Davies MJ, Woolf N, Robertson NB. Pathology of acute myocardial infarction with particular reference to occlusive coronary thrombi. Br Heart J 1976; 38: 659–64

3. Bertrand ME, Lefebure JM, Laine CL. Coronary angiography in acute transmural myocardial infarction. Am Heart J 1979; 97: 61–9

4. DeWood MA, Spores J, Notske R, et al. Prevalence of total coronary occlusion during the early hours of transmural myocardial infarction. N Engl J Med 1980; 303: 897–902

5. Falk E. Plaque rupture with severe pre-existing stenosis precipitating coronary thrombosis. Characteristics of coronary atherosclerotic plaques underlying fatal occlusive thrombi. Br Heart J 1983; 50: 127–34

6. Tennant R, Wiggers CJ. The effects of coronary occlusion on myocardial contraction. Am J Physiol 1935; 112: 351–61

7. Reimer KA, Lowe JE, Rasmussen MM, Jennings RB. The wavefront phenomenon of ischaemic cell death. 1. Myocardial infarct size vs duration of coronary occlusion in dogs. Circulation 1977; 56: 786–94

8. Yellon DM, Hearse DJ, Crome R, Wyse RKH. Temporal and spatial characteristics of evolving cell injury during regional myocardial ischemia in the dog: the 'borderline zone' controversy. J Am Coll Cardiol 1983; 2: 661–70

9. White HD, Norris RM, Brown MA, et al. Effects of intravenous streptokinase on left ventricular function and early survival after acute myocardial infarction. N Engl J Med 1987; 317: 850–5

10. Ohman EM, Califf RM, Topol EJ, et al. Consequences of reocclusion after successful reperfusion therapy in acute myocardial infarction. TAMI Study Group. Circulation 1990; 82: 781–91

11. Fletcher AP, Alkjaersig N, Smyrniotis FE, et al. Treatment of patients suffering from early myocardial infarction with massive and prolonged streptokinase therapy. Trans Assoc Am Phys 1958; 71: 287–96

12. Chazov EI, Matveeva LS, Mazaev AV, Sargin KE, Sadovskaia GV, Ruda MI. Acute myocardial infarction: intracoronary administration of fibrinolysis in acute myocardial infarction. Ter Arkh 1976; 48: 8–19

13. Rentrop KP, Blanke H, Karsch KR, et al. Acute myocardial infarction: intracoronary applications of nitroglycerin and streptokinase. Clin Cardiol 1979; 2: 354–63

14. Gruppo Italiano per lo Studio della Streptochinasi nell'Infarto Miocardico. Effectiveness of intravenous thrombolytic treatment in acute myocardial infarction. Lancet 1986; 1: 397–402

15. ISIS-2 (Second International Study of Infarct Survival) Collaborative Group. Randomised trial of intravenous streptokinase, oral aspirin, both or neither among 17,187 cases of suspected acute myocardial infarction: ISIS-2. Lancet 1988; 2: 349–60

16. AIMS Trial Study Group. Effect of intravenous APSAC on mortality after acute myocardial infarction: preliminary report of a placebo-controlled clinical trial. Lancet 1988; 1: 545–9

17. Wilcox RG, Von der Lippe G, Olsson CG, Jensen G, Skene AM, Hampton JR. Trial of tissue plasminogen activator for mortality reduction in acute myocardial infarction. Anglo-Scandinavian Study of Early Thrombolysis (ASSET). Lancet 1988; 2: 525–30

18. Fibrinolytic Therapy Trialists' (FTT) Collaborative Group. Indications for fibrinolytic therapy in suspected acute myocardial infarction: collaborative overview of early mortality and major morbidity results from all randomised trials of more than 1000 patients. Lancet 1994; 343: 311–22

19. Franzosi MG, Santoro E, De Vita C, et al. Ten-year follow-up of the first megatrial testing thromboloytic therapy in patients with acute myocardial infarction. Results of the Gruppo Italiano per lo Studio della Sopravvivenza nell'Infarcto-1 Study. Circulation 1998; 98: 2659–65

20. Sabatine MS, Cannon CP, Gibson CM, et al. Addition of clopidogrel to aspirin and fibrinolytic therapy for myocardial infarction with ST-segment elevation. N Engl J Med 2005; 352: 1179–89

21. Neuhaus KL, Von Essen R, Tebbe U, et al. Improved thrombolysis in acute myocardial infarction with front-loaded administration of alteplase: results of the rt-PA-APSAC patency study (TAPS). J Am Coll Cardiol 1992; 19: 885–91

22. The GUSTO Investigators. An international randomised trial comparing four thrombolytic strategies for acute myocardial infarction. N Engl J Med 1993; 329: 673–82

23. INJECT Study Group. International Joint Efficacy Comparison of Thrombolytics. Randomised, double-blind comparison of Reteplase double-bolus administration with streptokinase in acute myocardial infarction (INJECT): a trial to investigate equivalence. Lancet 1995; 346: 329–36

24. The Global Use of Strategies to Open Occluded Coronary Arteries (GUSTO III) Investigators. A comparison of reteplase with alteplase for acute myocardial infarction. N Engl J Med 1997; 337: 1118–23

25. The InTime-II Investigators. Intravenous n-PA for the treatment of infarcting myocardium early: InTime-II, a double-blind comparison of single-bolus lanoteplase vs accelerated alteplase for the treatment of patients with acute myocardial infarction. Eur Heart J 2000; 21: 2005–13

26. Assessment of the Safety and Efficacy of a New Thrombolytic Investigators. Single bolus tenecteplase compared with front-loaded alteplase in acute myocardial infarction: the ASSENT-2 double-blind randomised trial. Lancet 1999; 354: 716–22

27. The GUSTO Angiographic Investigators. The effects of tissue plasminogen activator, streptokinase, or both on coronary artery patency, ventricular function and survival after acute myocardial infarction. N Engl J Med 1993; 329: 1615–22

28. Meijer A, Verheugt FW, Werter CJ, Lie KI, Van der Pol JM, Van Eenige MJ. Aspirin versus coumadin in the prevention of reocclusion and recurrent ischaemia after successful

thrombolysis: a prospective placebo-controlled angiographic study. Results of the APRI-COT Study. Circulation 1993; 87: 1524–30

29. Rawles J. Halving of mortality at 1 year by domiciliary thrombolysis in the Grampian Region Early Anistreplase Trial (GREAT). J Am Coll Cardiol 1994; 23: 1–5

30. Ito M, Tomooka T, Sakai N, et al. A lack of myocardial perfusion immediately after successful thrombolysis: a predictor of poor recovery of left ventricular function in anterior myocardial infarction. Circulation 1992; 85: 1699–1705

31. Maes A, Van der Werf F, Nuyts J, et al. Impaired myocardial tissue perfusion early after successful thrombolysis. Impact on myocardial flow, metabolism and function at late follow up. Circulation 1995; 92: 2072–8

32. Gibson CM, Cannon CP, Murphy SA, et al. Relationship of TIMI Myocardial Perfusion Grade to mortality after administration of thrombolytic drugs. Circulation 2000; 101: 125–30

33. Verma S, Fedak P, Weisel R, et al. Fundamentals of reperfusion injury for the clinical cardiologist. Circulation 2002; 105: 2332–6

34. Giugliano RP, McCabe CH, Antman EM, et al. The Thrombolysis in Myocardial infarction (TIMI) investigators. Lower dose heparin with fibrinolysis is associated with lower rates of intracranial haemorrhage. Am Heart J 2001; 141: 742–50

35. Simoons ML, Maggioni AP, Knatterud G, et al. Individual risk assessment for intracranial haemorrhage during thrombolytic therapy. Lancet 1993; 342: 1523–8

36. Squire IB, Lawley W, Fletcher S, et al. Humoral and cellular responses up to 7.5 years after administration of streptokinase for acute myocardial infarction. Eur Heart J 1999; 20: 1245–52

37. Jennings K. Antibodies to streptokinase. Br Med J 1996; 312: 393–4

38. Schröder R, Dissman R, Brüggermann T, Wegscheider K, Linderer T, Tebbe U. Extent of early ST segment elevation resolution: a simple but strong predictor of outcome in patients with acute myocardial infarction. J Am Coll Cardiol 1994; 24: 384–91

39. Schröder R, Wegscheider K, Schröder K, Dissmann R, Meyer-Sabellek, for the INJECT Trial Group. Extent of early ST segment elevation resolution: a strong predictor of outcome in patients with acute myocardial infarction and a sensitive measure to compare thrombolytic regimes. J Am Coll Cardiol 1995; 26: 1657–64

40. Barbash GI, Birnbaum Y, Bogaerts K, et al. Treatment of reinfarction after thrombolytic therapy for acute myocardial infarction: an analysis of outcome and treatment choices in the global utilisation of streptokinase and tissue plasminogen activator for occluded coronary arteries (GUSTO-1) and assessment of the safety of a new thrombolytic (ASSENT-2) studies. Circulation 2001; 103: 954–60

41. Pitt B, Remme W, Zannad F, et al. Eplerenone, a selective aldosterone blocker, in patients with left ventricular dysfunction after myocardial infarction. N Engl J Med 2003; 348: 1309–21

42. Villella A, Maggioni AP, Villella M, et al., on behalf of the GISSI-2 Investigators. Prognostic significance of maximal exercise testing after myocardial infarction treated with thrombolytic agents: the GISSI-2 data-base. Lancet 1995; 346: 523–9

43. Madsen JK, Grande P, Saunamaki K, et al. Danish Multicenter Randomised Study of Invasive Versus Conservative Treatment in Patients with Inducible Ischemia After Thrombolysis in Acute Myocardial Infarction (DANAMI). Circulation 1997; 96: 748–55

44. Fernandez-Aviles F, Alonso JJ, Castro-Beira A, et al. Routine invasive strategy within 2 hours of thrombolysis versus ischaemia-guided conservative approach for acute myocardial infarction with ST-segment elevation (GRACIA-1): a randomised controlled trial. Lancet 2004; 364: 1045–53

45. Thiemann DR, Coresh J, Schulman P, et al. Lack of benefit of intravenous thrombolysis in patients with myocardial infarction who are older than 75 years. Circulation 2000; 101: 2239–46

46. Boersma E, Maas AC, Deckers JW, Simoons ML. Early thrombolytic treatment in acute myocardial infarction: reappraisal of the golden hour. Lancet 1996; 348: 771–5

47. Keeley EC, Boura JA, Grimes CL. Primary angioplasty versus intravenous thrombolytic therapy for acute myocardial infarction: a quantitative review of 23 randomised trials. Lancet 2003; 361: 13–20

48. Dalby M, Bouzamondo A, Lechat P, Montalescot G. Transfer for primary angioplasty versus immediate thrombolysis in acute myocardial infarction: a meta-analysis. Circulation 2003; 108: 1809–14

49. Nallamothu BK, Bates ER. Percutaneous coronary intervention versus fibrinolytic therapy in acute myocardial infarction: is timing (almost) everything? Am J Cardiol 2003; 92: 824–6

50. Steg PG, Bonnefoy E, Chabaud S, et al., for the Comparison of Angioplasty and Prehospital Thrombolysis in Acute Myocardial Infarction (CAPTIM) Investigators. Impact of time to treatment on mortality after prehospital fibrinolysis or primary angioplasty: data from the CAPTIM randomised clinical trial. Circulation 2003; 108: 2851–6

51. Widimsky P, Bucleskinsky T, Vorac D, et al. Long distance transport for primary angioplasty versus immediate thrombolysis in acute myocardial infarction: final results of the randomised national multicentre trial – PRAGUE-2. Eur Heart J 2003; 24: 94–104

52. The Task Force on the Management of Acute Myocardial Infarction of the European Society of Cardiology. Management of acute myocardial infarction in patients presenting with ST-segment elevation. Eur Heart J 2003; 24: 28–66

53. Hillegass WB, Jollis GJ, Granger CB, Ohman EM, Califf RM, Mark DB. Intracranial hemorrhage risk and new thrombolytic therapies in acute myocardial infarction. Am J Cardiol 1994; 73: 444–9

54. Weaver WD. The role of thrombolytic drugs in the management of myocardial infarction. Comparative clinical trials. Eur Heart J 1996; 17 (Suppl F): 9–15

55. Rogers WJ, Canto JG, Lambrew CT, et al., for the Investigators in the National Registry of Myocardial Infarction 1, 2 and 3. Temporal trends in the treatment of over 1.5 million patients with myocardial infarction in the US from 1990 through 1999. J Am Coll Cardiol 2000; 36: 2056–63

56. Grimes CL, DeMaria AN. Optimal utilisation of thrombolytic therapy for acute myocardial infarction: concepts and controversies. J Am Coll Cardiol 1990; 16: 223–31

57. Norris RM, on behalf of the UK Heart Attack Study Investigators. Sudden cardiac death and acute myocardial infarction in three British Health Districts: the UK Heart Attack Study. London: Education Committee of the British Heart Foundation, 1999

4

Primary coronary intervention for acute myocardial infarction

Felix Zijlstra

Timely restoration of antegrade coronary blood flow in the infarct-related artery of a patient with acute myocardial infarction results in myocardial salvage and improved survival.[1,2] Intravenous thrombolytic therapy and immediate cardiac catheterization, followed by primary coronary intervention (PCI), are both widely used reperfusion therapies. A recent review of 23 randomized trials comparing these two treatment modalities favors PCI with regard to mortality, reinfarction and stroke.[3] Given the superior safety and efficacy of PCI, this treatment is now preferred when logistics allow this approach, even when this necessitates additional transportation.[4] As had been shown for PCI therapy for stable and unstable angina, it is likely that the results from various hospitals may differ considerably.[5,6] Establishing and maintaining a proficient PCI program takes great institutional will and effort, and even institutions with a large experience in angioplasty for stable and unstable angina will have something of a learning curve for PCI.

PRIMARY CORONARY INTERVENTION IN PATIENTS INELIGIBLE FOR THROMBOLYTIC THERAPY

Starting in the early 1980s, case series have reported the successful use of balloon angioplasty without concomitant administration of thrombolytic therapy, in a wide range of clinical presentations of patients with myocardial infarction, including cardiogenic shock, after prior bypass surgery and in patients with contraindications to thrombolytic therapy.[7,8] In a post-hoc analysis of the Primary Angioplasty in Myocardial Infarction (PAMI) trial, patients with relative thrombolytic contraindications, such as late presentation, age > 70 years, or prior bypass surgery, constituted a high-risk group with significant morbidity and mortality after thrombolysis. Both in-hospital (3% vs. 13%, $p = 0.025$) and 6 months' mortality (3% vs. 16%, $p = 0.009$) were lower with primary angioplasty.[9] In the Medicine versus Angiography in Thrombolytic Exclusion (MATE) trial, 201 patients with suspected acute myocardial infarction, ineligible for thrombolysis, were enrolled in a prospective randomized trial. Patients were randomized to early triage angiography and subsequent therapies based on the angiogram versus conventional medical therapy. In the invasive group 98% had angiography and 58% underwent revascularization, whereas in the conservative group 60% subsequently underwent non-protocol angiography and 37% received revascularization. The primary endpoint of death or recurrent ischemic events favored the invasive group (13% vs. 34%, p = 0.0002). However, at a median follow-up of 21 months, no differences in late revascularization, reinfarction or all-cause mortality were apparent.[10]

Patients with a non-diagnostic electrocardiogram

The relative merits of an invasive versus a conservative strategy in patients with non-ST elevation myocardial infarction were explored by the Myocardial Infarction Triage and Intervention (MITI) investigators. In a patient with suspected acute myocardial ischemia or infarction, a non-diagnostic electrocardiogram is usually followed by conservative therapy in hospitals that depend on thrombolysis as reperfusion therapy. If clinical suspicion is high, a non-diagnostic electrocardiogram (no ST elevation) may be followed by triage angiography in hospitals with an active primary angioplasty program. In this MITI cohort of 1635 consecutive patients with symptoms of acute infarction without ST elevation, 308 patients were presented to hospitals whose initial strategy favored early angiography and intervention, versus 1327 similar patients who presented to hospitals that favor a conservative initial approach. Triage angiography occurred in 59% vs. 8% (p < 0.001) and angioplasty was performed in 45% vs. 6% (p < 0.001). The early invasive strategy resulted in a lower short-term and 4-year mortality: 20% vs. 37%, p < 0.001. Multivariate analysis showed a significantly lower long-term mortality with a hazard ratio of 0.61 (95% confidence interval 0.47–0.80), in patients admitted to hospitals favoring an invasive strategy.[11] In a randomized comparison of early invasive and conservative strategies in patients with unstable coronary syndromes, 833 of 2220 (38%) patients without ST elevation presented with enzymatic evidence of acute myocardial infarction. The benefits of an invasive approach found in these acute coronary syndrome patients were most pronounced in the large sub-group presenting with acute myocardial infarction and a 'non-diagnostic electrocardiogram'.[12]

Presentation after the conventional reperfusion time window

Late presentation may be a reason to withhold reperfusion therapy, in particular thrombolysis. Data from the Treatment with Enoxapam and Tirofiban in Acute Myocardial Infarction (TETAMI) registry and randomized trial give a clear picture of the magnitude of this specific problem in routine clinical practice. From a cohort of 2737 patients who presented with ST elevation or a new left bundle branch block, 1654 (60%) presented at < 12 h after the onset of symptoms. Reperfusion therapy was given to 1196 (72%) of these 1654 patients; 458 (28%) were deemed 'ineligible' for reperfusion, mostly because of contraindications to thrombolysis. From the entire cohort, 1083 (40%) presented > 12 h after symptom onset, and only 34 (3%) received reperfusion therapy.[13] In response to these rather sobering facts it is clear that we should intensify our efforts to provide initial diagnosis and therapy for acute myocardial infarction in the early hours after the onset of symptoms.

Patients with contraindications to thrombolysis

Out of 5869 patients with acute myocardial infarction registered by the Maximal Individual Therapy in Acute Myocardial Infarction (MITRA) trial, 337 (6%) patients had at least one strong contraindication to thrombolysis. Out of these 337 patients 46 (15%) were treated with primary angioplasty, and 276 (85%) were treated conservatively. Hospital mortality was significantly lower in patients who received primary angioplasty: 2% vs. 25% ($p = 0.001$), with an odds ratio for death after multivariate analysis of 0.46 ($p = 0.02$).[14] The clinical outcome after conservative management of patients with acute ST segment elevation myocardial infarction and contraindications to thrombolysis has been described in the 1 799 704 patients enrolled between June 1994 and January 2003 in the National Registry of Myocardial Infarction. A total of 19 917 patients had thrombolytic contraindications and were potential candidates for triage angiography and immediate revascularization. The in-hospital mortality rate in non-revascularized patients was 31%, confirming the very high-risk nature of this clinical condition. In-hospital mortality with revascularization was 11%, a risk reduction of 64%. This treatment effect remained significant after propensity analysis and following a second logistic model: odds ratio 0.64, 95% confidence interval 0.56–0.75.[15] Given this abundance of circumstantial evidence, it is clear that an invasive approach must be strongly recommended in a broad spectrum of patients presenting with suspected myocardial infarction, especially in patients who are ineligible for thrombolytic therapy.

PRIMARY CORONARY INTERVENTION IN PATIENTS ELIGIBLE FOR THROMBOLYTIC THERAPY

Several quantitative overviews and/or meta-analyses of randomized controlled trials comparing primary coronary interventions with thrombolytic therapy in thrombolysis-eligible patients have consistently shown that primary coronary intervention results in a lower rate of death, stroke and reinfarction. However, it has been argued that almost none of these trials have used prehospital lytic therapy instead of in-hospital initiated thrombolysis therapy. One report from the Primary Coronary Angioplasty versus Thrombolysis (PCAT) trialists collaborative group shows the relative time independence of clinical outcome after primary coronary intervention.[16] Event rates at 30 days in 6763 patients enrolled in 22 randomized controlled trials according to treatment allocation are presented in Table 4.1. Overall, 7.9% of patients randomized to thrombolysis died within 30 days, compared to 5.3% of those randomized to primary coronary intervention. Even in patients with a very short presentation delay, intervention resulted in a markedly lower rate of death as well the combination of death and reinfarction.

Table 4.1 Adverse events, death and reinfarction at 30 days in 6763 patients enrolled in 22 randomized controlled trials, stratified for time from symptom onset to randomization

	< 1 h	1–2 h	2–3 h	3–6 h	> 6 h
Thrombolysis	14.9	10.4	13.6	15.0	17.6
PCI	6.1	6.8	7.4	7.2	10.3

PCI, primary coronary intervention

THE MAIN ISSUES PERTINENT TO THE DELIVERY OF PERCUTANEOUS CORONARY INTERVENTION THERAPY FOR ACUTE MYOCARDIAL INFARCTION

Prehospital phase

A speedy response and early recognition of acute myocardial infarction by general practitioners and ambulance services are of great importance, mainly for two reasons. First, mortality in the very early hours is substantial, and many patients die before adequate medical help has been sought and delivered.[17] Second, although the results of PCI therapy are less time-dependent than the results of thrombolysis, in particular during the first few hours, time is muscle.[18] Confirmation of the diagnosis of acute myocardial infarction by 12-lead electrocardiography, by either general practitioners or ambulance paramedics, allows a substantial reduction of the time delay to first balloon inflation, because the hospital and the catheterization laboratory can be prepared in advance, and the emergency room and the coronary care unit (CCU) (with their unavoidable delays) can be skipped on the way to acute angiography.[19] Furthermore, it is an important opportunity to start initial pharmacological therapy, and use the transportation time in this regard.[20–23] A PCI center must therefore develop additional specific training programs for general practitioners and ambulance services. Excellent communication with these first-line providers of care for patients with acute myocardial infarction is of paramount importance, as this will be among the main factors determining time to therapy.

The first 15 in-hospital minutes

If a definitive diagnosis has not been made before arrival at the hospital, it is very important that additional delays are avoided. A limited history and physical examination should be performed and a 12-lead electrocardiogram should be made and interpreted within 5–10 min.[17] Blood may be drawn for tests, but results should not be waited for; a chest X-ray is unnecessary. The first responsibility of the emergency room physician is to contact the catheterization laboratory and to get the patient there as soon as possible.

Finally, a flexible attitude shared by the catheterization laboratory staff and interventional cardiologist is a prerequisite. They should be prepared to change their program at a moment's notice, drop an elective case planned for intracoronary ultrasound, multiple stenting, etc., or get out of bed in the middle of the night, to do this job as quickly and proficiently as they can.

Initial pharmacological therapy

Adequate pain relief and supplemental oxygen are essential, not only for humanitarian reasons, but in particular because the patient has to endure angiography and angioplasty.[17] Aspirin should be given, at least 300 mg soluble chewable, but as gastrointestinal symptoms are frequent, it may be preferable to give 500 mg of aspirin intravenously. Sublingual and intravenous nitroglycerine as well as intravenous β-blockers,[20] unless contraindicated, should be given in an effort to lower oxygen consumption and alleviate myocardial ischemia. Intravenous heparin can be used in an attempt to increase initial patency rates of the infarct-related vessel,[21] and plays an important role during the percutaneous coronary intervention. Abciximab or tirofiban as pretreatment and as concomitant therapy can be recommended for most patients.[22,23] Clopidogrel is now used in all patients with an acute coronary syndrome, and should be started with a loading dose of at least 300 mg.[24]

Angiography

Vascular access can be obtained by either the femoral or the radial approach, but the former is generally preferred. Femoral access allows larger devices if necessary (intra-aortic balloon pump)[25] or transvenous pacing when indicated. The physician can choose between 5, 6 or 7Fr sheaths and catheters. The advantage of the radial approach is the low risk of bleeding complications.

An angiogram of the non-infarcted artery should be performed first to allow identification of multivessel disease and collateral flow into the infarct zone. Contrast ventriculography is necessary only to help determine the infarcted artery if this is uncertain, based on information of the electrocardiogram and the coronary angiogram, and can usually be skipped. In general, angiography of the infarct artery is performed with a guiding catheter, 6Fr, to be able to proceed immediately with PCI if indicated. During this phase the interventional cardiologist must try to give answers to the following questions:

1. Can I identify the infarct artery with certainty and will I be able to get it open? (If not, ask for help; don't try to be a hero.)

2. Consider a conservative approach when there is spontaneous reperfusion, a small myocardial territory at risk, or extensive collateral circulation and think about this: does this patient need bypass surgery, either acutely or following initial stabilization?

3. If the decision to go for PCI is taken:

   Do I need venous access? Temporary pacing? Intra-aortic balloon pumping? In particular, during recanalization of right coronary arteries, bradycardia and hypotension may develop that may necessitate large amounts of intravenous fluids and 0.5–2.0 mg atropine or even pressure therapy. The interventional cardiologist who is not prepared to handle these types of complications, but lets him/herself be surprised by these sudden events, may lose a patient.

PCI procedure

After completion of the angiographic study and with a clear concept on what should be done, the infarct artery should be crossed with a soft, floppy steerable guidewire. After passing the wire it is often possible to have a first impression of the distal vessel following intracoronary nitrates. Final balloon and/or stent sizing should be adequate, around 1–1.1:1 balloon to artery ratio. This mandates repeated bolus doses of intracoronary nitrates after initial restoration of flow, in order to avoid serious underestimation of the true arterial size. Initial reperfusion can usually be obtained with one or two balloon inflations at 8–12 atm. Optimal angiographic visualization of the lesion and the distal vessel in multiple projections is necessary, to assess the result and define the need for further balloon inflations and stenting. The operator should strive for an optimal result with < 20% residual luminal narrowing and TIMI 3 flow as well as evidence of myocardial reperfusion.[26] Most operators prefer to place a stent, to cover or seal the ruptured plaque, although all trials reported to date have enrolled selected patients after initial angiography. In selected patients, stenting with a drug-eluting stent may be preferable, to prevent restenosis and late additional target vessel revascularization.[27]

With regard to stenting it should be noted that almost all sudden occlusions of infarct arteries after 'plain old balloon angioplasty' occur in-hospital and can usually be managed, but subacute stent thrombosis, although rare, may occur after discharge with sometimes dramatic consequences. This may in particular be the case with some of the drug-eluting stents. All stented patients should be treated with aspirin and clopidogrel for at least 9 months.[24]

Risk stratification and further management

When the care of patients with an acute myocardial infarction is placed into the hands of interventional cardiologists it is crucial that they pay as meticulous attention to further management as to the initial procedure. Therefore, some of the most important aspects are briefly delineated here. Based on the available clinical data, the angiographic findings and the 12-lead electrocardiogram,[26,28–30] after the PCI procedure the risk to the individual patient can be estimated reliably and further management can be tailored accordingly. In high-risk patients, intra-aortic balloon pumping may be considered.[25] During the first days it is appropriate to assess left ventricular function by echocardiography or radionuclide ventriculography.[17] Most patients have early sheath removal 0–3 h after the PCI procedure. The use of a closure device can be of benefit for patient and nursing staff. Two to three days of low molecular weight heparin is appropriate. Angiotensin converting enzyme inhibition is given to patients with depressed left ventricular function, and patients should have diet counseling and start with cholesterol-lowering therapy.[17] In particular, as patients now are discharged after 2–4 days,[29] the outpatient rehabilitation program has become a very important and integral part of infarct patient management, including many aspects of secondary prevention such as smoking cessation and weight reduction.

In patients with multivessel disease, the need for additional revascularization procedures should be addressed. Signs and symptoms of recurrent ischemia must be carefully sought for during the few in-hospital days and in particular during visits to the outpatient clinic. Dependent on the setting, the general practitioner of the patient may play a central role in this monitoring process.

The most important aspects of PCI for acute myocardial infarction are summarized in the following ten rules:

1. In suspected myocardial infarction, initial assessment < 15 min: TIME = MUSCLE = LIVES.

2. When diagnosis of myocardial infarction is confirmed before hospital arrival, go to catheterization laboratory, and not to emergency room or CCU.

3. Do not forget aspirin, clopidogrel, glycoprotein II-b III-a inhibitors, heparin, nitrates and a β-blocker.

4. Visualize both coronary arteries.

5. Consider conservative management and acute or elective coronary artery bypass graft.

6. Use a balloon and a stent; forget other techniques.

7. Be sure that somebody looks after the patient when you perform angiography and PCI.

8. Beware of, and prepare for, reperfusion arrhythmias, bradycardia and hypotension.

9. Do not undersize.

10. Stent the plaque, not the vessel.

Two of the many patients admitted to our hospital on Easter Saturday 2004 will illustrate many of the discussed issues of the modern care of patients with acute myocardial infarctions (Figures 4.1 and 4.2).

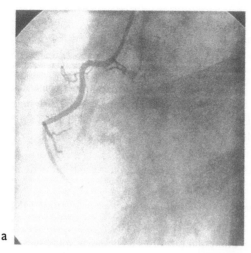

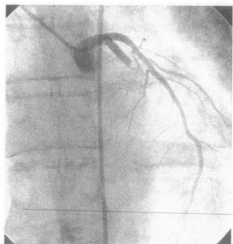

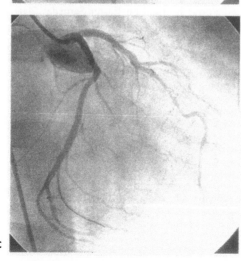

Figure 4.1 A 53-year-old man experienced the sudden onset of crushing chest pain at 18.30. An ambulance was called and arrived at 19.20, and found a patient in severe respiratory distress, with a systolic blood pressure of 60 mmHg. A 12-lead electrocardiogram showed a sinus rhythm of 100 beats per minute, with ST elevation in inferior and lateral leads and ST depression in anterior leads. Fluids and aspirin were given intravenously and O_2 therapy was started using a mask. During emergency transportation, atropine and epinephrine (adrenaline) were given for bradycardia and absence of measurable blood pressure. The patient came into the catheterization laboratory at 20.30 in profound shock and respiratory failure. Arterial blood gas analysis showed a pH of 7.1, pO_2 5.6 kPa and pCO_2 6.2 kPa. An anesthesiologist was asked to place the patient on mechanical ventilation, while coronary angiography was performed. The right coronary artery was a small non-dominant vessel (a), the left coronary artery showed a total occlusion of the proximal circumflex artery (b) and a left anterior descending artery with bridging, but no signs of significant coronary artery disease. After passage of a wire, a stent was placed with immediate restoration of antegrade flow in this very large artery that supplied the entire lateral, posterior and inferior wall of the left ventricle (c). An intra-aortic balloon pump and a pulmonary artery catheter were placed, and the patient went to the intensive care unit at 22.00.

The hemodynamic situation stabilized within a few hours and detubation followed the next day. On day 3 the balloon pump was removed and the patient made an excellent clinical recovery.

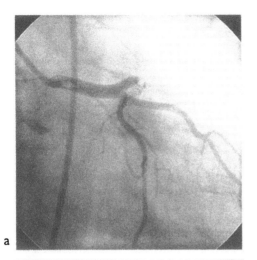

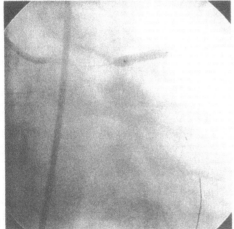

Figure 4.2 A 58-year-old woman with diabetes did not feel well and experienced mild dyspnea around 22.00. Although her symptoms continued, she fell asleep and woke up 5–6 h later, when she still experienced identical symptoms. Following a telephone consultation of her general practitioner, an ambulance arrived at 04.20. A 12-lead electrocardiogram showed sinus rhythm, 76 beats per minute, with pathological Q-waves and ST elevation in V1–V4. Following the administration of aspirin, clopidogrel and heparin, she was transferred to the catheterization laboratory, where she arrived at 05.00. Coronary angiography showed an occluded left anterior descending artery (a), that was dilated and stented (b), with an excellent result (c).

The patient was discharged on day 3, with aspirin, clopidogrel, metoprolol, enalapril, insulin and a statin and was enrolled in a cardiac rehabilitation program.

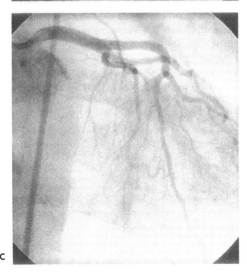

REFERENCES

1. The GUSTO Investigators. An international randomized trial comparing four thrombolytic strategies for acute myocardial infarction. N Engl J Med 1993; 329: 673–82

2. The GUSTO Angiographic Investigators. The effects of tissue plasminogen activator, streptokinase, or both on coronary-artery patency, ventricular function, and survival after acute myocardial infarction. N Engl J Med 1993; 329: 1615–22

3. Keeley EC, Boura JA, Grines CL. Primary angioplasty versus intravenous thrombolytic therapy for acute myocardial infarction: a quantitative review of 23 randomised trials. Lancet 2003; 361: 13–20

4. Zijlstra F. Angioplasty vs thrombolysis for acute myocardial infarction: a quantitative overview of the effects of interhospital transportation. Eur Heart J 2003; 24: 21–3

5. Magid DJ, Calonge BN, Rumsfeld JS, et al.; National Registry of Myocardial Infarction 2 and 3 Investigators. Relation between hospital primary angioplasty volume and mortality for patients with acute MI treated with primary angioplasty vs thrombolytic therapy. J Am Med Assoc 2000; 284: 3131–8

6. Canto JG, Every NR, Magid DJ, et al.; National Registry of Myocardial Infarction 2 Investigators. The volume of primary angioplasty procedures and survival after acute myocardial infarction. N Engl J Med 2000; 342: 1573–80

7. Hartzler GO, Rutherford BD, McConahay DR, et al. Percutaneous transluminal coronary angioplasty with and without thrombolytic therapy for treatment of acute myocardial infarction. Am Heart J 1983; 106: 965–73

8. O'Keefe JH Jr, Bailey WL, Rutherford BD, Hartzler GO. Primary angioplasty for acute myocardial infarction in 1,000 consecutive patients. Results in an unselected population and high-risk subgroups. Am J Cardiol 1993; 72: 107G–15G

9. Stone GW, Grines CL, Browne KF, et al.; Primary Angioplasty in Myocardial Infarction (PAMI) Investigators. Outcome of different reperfusion strategies in patients with former contraindications to thrombolytic therapy: a comparison of primary angioplasty and tissue plasminogen activator. Cathet Cardiovasc Diagn 1996; 39: 333–9

10. McCullough PA, O'Neill WW, Graham M, et al. A prospective randomized trial of triage angiography in acute coronary syndromes ineligible for thrombolytic therapy. Results of the medicine versus angiography in thrombolytic exclusion (MATE) trial. J Am Coll Cardiol 1998; 32: 596–605

11. Scull GS, Martin JS, Weaver WD, Every NR. MITI Investigators. Myocardial Infarction Triage and Intervention. Early angiography versus conservative treatment in patients with non-ST elevation acute myocardial infarction. J Am Coll Cardiol 2000; 35: 895–902

12. Cannon CP, Weintraub WS, Demopoulos LA, et al.; Thrombolysis in Myocardial Infarction 18 Investigators. TACTICS (Treat Angina with Aggrastat and Determine Cost of Therapy with an Invasive or Conservative Strategy). Comparison of early invasive and conservative strategies in patients with unstable coronary syndromes treated with the glycoprotein IIb/IIIa inhibitor tirofiban. N Engl J Med 2001; 344: 1879–87

13. Cohen M, Gensini GF, Maritz F, et al.; TETAMI Investigators. Prospective evaluation of clinical outcomes after acute ST-elevation myocardial infarction in patients who are ineligible for reperfusion therapy: preliminary results from the TETAMI registry and randomized trial. Circulation 2003; 108 (Suppl 1): III14–21

14. Zahn R, Schuster S, Schiele R, et al.; Maximal Individual Therapy in Acute Myocardial Infarction (MITRA) Study Group. Comparison of primary angioplasty with conservative therapy in patients with acute myocardial infarction and contraindications for thrombolytic therapy. Cathet Cardiovasc Interv 1999; 46: 127–33

15. Grzybowski M, Clements EA, Parsons L, et al. Mortality benefit of immediate revascularization of acute ST-segment elevation myocardial infarction in patients with

contraindications to thrombolytic therapy: a propensity analysis. J Am Med Assoc 2003; 290: 1891–8

16. Zijlstra F, Patel A, Jones M, et al. Clinical characteristics and outcome of patients with early (< 2 h), intermediate (2–4 h) and late (> 4 h) presentation treated by primary coronary angioplasty or thrombolytic therapy for acute myocardial infarction. Eur Heart J 2002; 23: 550–7

17. The Task Force on the Management of Acute Myocardial Infarction of the European Society of Cardiology. Acute myocardial infarction: prehospital and in-hospital management. Eur Heart J 1996; 17: 43–63

18. De Luca G, Suryapranata H, Ottervanger JP, Antman EM. Time delay to treatment and mortality in primary angioplasty for acute myocardial infarction: every minute of delay counts. Circulation 2004; 109: 1223–5

19. Zijlstra F. Long-term benefit of primary angioplasty compared to thrombolytic therapy for acute myocardial infarction. Eur Heart J 2000; 21: 1487–9

20. Halkin A, Grines CL, Cox DA, et al. Impact of intravenous beta-blockade before primary angioplasty on survival in patients undergoing mechanical reperfusion therapy for acute myocardial infarction. J Am Coll Cardiol 2004; 43: 1780–7

21. Zijlstra F, Ernst N, de Boer MJ, et al. Influence of prehospital administration of aspirin and heparin on initial patency of the infarct-related artery in patients with acute ST elevation myocardial infarction. J Am Coll Cardiol 2002; 39: 1733–7

22. Montalescot G, Barragan P, Wittenberg O, et al.; ADMIRAL Investigators. Abciximab before direct angioplasty and stenting in myocardial infarction regarding acute and long-term follow-up. Platelet glycoprotein IIb/IIIa inhibition with coronary stenting for acute myocardial infarction. N Engl J Med 2001; 344: 1895–903

23. Van't Hof AW, Ernst N, de Boer MJ, et al.; On-TIME study group. Facilitation of primary coronary angioplasty by early start of a glycoprotein 2b/3a inhibitor: results of the ongoing tirofiban in myocardial infarction evaluation (On-TIME) trial. Eur Heart J 2004; 25: 837–46

24. Mehta SR, Yusuf S, Peters RJ, et al.; Clopidogrel in Unstable angina to prevent Recurrent Events trial (CURE) Investigators. Effects of pretreatment with clopidogrel and aspirin followed by long-term therapy in patients undergoing percutaneous coronary intervention: the PCI-CURE study. Lancet 2001; 358: 527–33

25. Stone GW, Ohman EM, Miller MF, et al. Contemporary utilization and outcomes of intra-aortic balloon counterpulsation in acute myocardial infarction: the benchmark registry. J Am Coll Cardiol 2003; 41: 1940–5

26. Henriques JP, Zijlstra F, van't Hof AW, et al. Angiographic assessment of reperfusion in acute myocardial infarction by myocardial blush grade. Circulation 2003; 107: 2115–19

27. Lemos PA, Saia F, Hofma SH, et al. Short- and long-term clinical benefit of sirolimus-eluting stents compared to conventional bare stents for patients with acute myocardial infarction. J Am Coll Cardiol 2004; 43: 704–8

28. Van't Hof AWJ, Liem AL, de Boer MJ, Zijlstra F, on behalf of the Zwolle Myocardial Infarction Study Group. Clinical value of 12-lead electrocardiogram after successful reperfusion therapy for acute myocardial infarction. Lancet 1997; 350: 615–19

29. De Luca G, Suryapranata H, van't Hof AW, et al. Prognostic assessment of patients with acute myocardial infarction treated with primary angioplasty: implications for early discharge. Circulation 2004; 109: 2737–43

30. Henriques JP, Zijlstra F; Zwolle Myocardial Infarction Study Group. Frequency and sequelae of ST elevation acute myocardial infarction caused by spontaneous distal embolization from unstable coronary lesions. Am J Cardiol 2003; 91: 708–11

5

Anti-platelet treatment in reperfusion therapy for acute myocardial infarction

Emilia Solinas, Gianluca Gonzi, Diego Ardissino

INTRODUCTION

Anti-platelet therapy is essential in reperfusion therapy for acute myocardial infarction, because it significantly reduces the incidence of major coronary events and ischemic complications. The therapeutic approach to coronary diseases concentrates on the pathophysiological mechanisms underlying intracoronary thrombosis, a process in which platelets play a pivotal role and which can be efficaciously controlled and prevented by anti-platelet therapy. Since acute myocardial infarction occurs in consequence of the rupture of an atherosclerotic plaque, leading to platelet activation, aggregation and subsequent thrombus formation with vessel occlusion, the most effective reperfusion regimen is the association of fibrinolytic therapy and platelet-inhibiting drugs.

This benefit was first demonstrated early in 1988 with the ISIS study, with a reduction of 35 days' mortality from 13.2% in patients with acute myocardial infarction (AMI) not receiving any reperfusion treatment or anti-platelet therapy, to 8% in patients treated with streptokinase plus aspirin. After this trial aspirin has become a cornerstone in the treatment of AMI.

Nonetheless, aspirin has many limitations, being first a relatively weak anti-platelet blocker, and second because, in up to 30% of persons, a condition of resistance to the drug can be found, affecting the extension of platelet activation and aggregation inhibition.

These findings have driven the development of new anti-platelet agents such as GP IIb/IIIa inhibitors, but the strategy of associating these potent anti-platelet agents with either a full dose or reduced dose fibrinolytic has shown only a modest reduction in the incidence of reinfarction, which has been largely offset by the concomitant increase of bleeding complications.

Among new anti-platelet agents, is clopidogrel, which is a more potent platelet inhibitor than aspirin, but less than GP IIb/IIIA. It has recently been shown that, for patients receiving fibrinolytic therapy, its association with aspirin is safe and effective.

Anti-platelet agents play a pivotal role in association with primary angioplasty, which represents the strategy of choice in the treatment of acute myocardial infarction.

PATHOGENESIS

The initial mechanism in the pathogenesis of acute coronary syndromes, which is responsible for starting the thrombotic process, is the fissuring and/or rupture of the atheromatous plaque, and the subsequent exposure of subendothelial collagen and the lipid core.[1,2] These components are potent stimulants of platelet activation and highly thrombogenic,[3] a process that leads to a reduction in coronary flow.

The interaction of platelets with the vessel wall, together with their contribution to the formation of the atheromatous plaque and the thrombotic process, play a major role in the pathogenesis of coronary disease. The integrity of the vascular endothelium is fundamental in preventing the onset and progression of vascular thrombosis, which is otherwise amplified by the endothelial wall damage due to atheromatous plaque rupture, the entry of thrombogenic substances into the blood flow, and the interaction of platelets with coagulation factors.

Endothelial damage leads to the immediate deposit of platelets on the damaged wall by means of a mechanism of adhesion to the various components of the subendothelial connective matrix, including fibrin, collagen and laminin.[4] This process of platelet adhesion is initially mediated by von Willebrand factor (vWF), a glycosylated multimeric protein that is synthesized by the endothelium and secreted into the subendothelium, where it binds to collagen. Other plasma factors, such as fibronectin, fibrinogen and thrombospondin, are also directly involved in the platelet adhesion mechanism. This adhesion essentially depends on specific membrane platelet glycoproteins. Glycoprotein IIb platelet receptors bind to vWF, the principal glycoprotein involved in the initial contact of platelets with the vessel wall. Platelet adhesion is also influenced by hemodynamic flow conditions: the presence of high wall shear stress potentiates platelet adhesion and subsequent activation.[5]

Platelet activation occurs after adhesion and may be induced by a large number of biochemical stimuli, the most powerful of which include the presence of thrombin and platelet adhesion to collagen and the other components of the subendothelial matrix.

After the platelets have adhered to the subendothelial matrix and have therefore been activated, they undergo a conformational modification that leads to the exposure of the previously unexpressed GP IIb/IIIa platelet receptors, and the simultaneous release of the various substances contained in the platelet granules (serotonin, thromboxane A_2, ADP, epinephrine), which are capable of activating additional platelets.

The common final pathway leading to the formation of a platelet thrombus is platelet aggregation. Further platelet recruitment depends on the exposure of the GP IIb/IIIa receptor, which is possible only after the conformational modifications undergone by previously activated platelets. This receptor mainly binds to fibrinogen, a key component of the aggregation process in so far as it determines the formation of molecular bridges between the GP IIb/IIIa receptors of adjacent platelets. This binds them together in a step that precedes thrombus formation and which progressively extends, as further platelets are recruited and activated. Unless it is controlled and regulated by compensatory mechanisms, this process may lead to the occlusion of the coronary lumen. This event is prevented by the anti-aggregant substances (prostacyclin, endothelium-derived relaxing factor (EDRF), nitric oxide (NO), ADPase) secreted by neighboring undamaged endothelial cells.[6]

However, the platelet thrombus is relatively unstable and causes only an initial obstruction of coronary flow. It is the endothelial damage that activates the coagulation cascade, which starts when tissue factor comes into contact with various circulating factors and ends with the formation of the fibrin that stabilizes the primary platelet thrombus. After its self-amplification, tissue factor forms an additional complex with factor X of the coagulation cascade on the surface of the activated platelets, whose membranes contain phospholipids capable of sustaining and potentiating the cascade by means of an intrinsic pathway. After its activation, factor X reassembles with complex V, but this is not capable of converting prothrombin into thrombin. The mechanism activating factor V (and therefore leading to the formation of thrombin) is not fully understood, but it is believed that a feedback mechanism allows moderate prothrombin levels to activate factor V which, by complexing with factor Xa, is capable of generating thrombin.[7] All of these reactions occur on the surfaces of activated platelets. Thrombin-mediated platelet activation can also be considered a positive feedback mechanism that increases thrombin levels and leads to thrombus formation. Thrombin plays a key role in the recruitment of additional platelets because it is *per se* the most potent physiological platelet activator.[8]

Thrombin subsequently catalyzes the conversion of fibrinogen to fibrin, a filamentous protein that can bind to other monomers in order to form a stratified reticulum capable of trapping blood cells: a fibrin thrombus.

ASPIRIN

Pharmacokinetics

Aspirin inhibits prostaglandin G/H synthase (PGHS), the cyclo-oxygenase enzyme that catalyzes the first step of the conversion of arachidonic acid to thromboxane A_2, one of the more than 90 substances inducing platelet aggregation. Two isozymes of PGHS are known: PGHS-1 is expressed in virtually all cells of the human body; and PGHS-2 is undetectable in most mammalian tissues, but its expression can be induced in monocytes, endothelial cells and other specialized cells in response to various inflammatory and mitogen mediators. The inhibition of PGHS by aspirin is permanent in platelets, because they are unable to generate new cyclo-oxygenase.

The mechanism of action of aspirin is related to a conformational change in the structure of the active site of PGHS. The carboxylic moiety of salicylic acid acetylates the hydroxyl group of a serine residue, at position 529, in the polypeptide chain of human platelet prostaglandin G/H synthase; when this happens the acetyl group protrudes into the cyclo-oxygenase channel at a critical site for arachidonic acid interaction with the tyrosine residue responsible for initiating catalysis.

Orally ingested aspirin is absorbed rapidly from the stomach and the upper small intestine primarily by passive diffusion of the non-dissociated lipid-soluble aspirin and in part as salicylate. The absorbed ester is rapidly hydrolyzed to salicylate in plasma, the liver, the lungs and erythrocytes. Salicylate is further metabolized mostly to salicyluric acid and partly to ester or acyl glucuronide. A small fraction is oxidized to gentisic acid and other metabolites without pharmacological effects. Salicylates are excreted mainly by the kidneys. The plasma half-life of aspirin is approximately 15 min while that of salicylate is dose dependent and ranges between 2 and 12 h.

A variable platelet response to aspirin has been described in patients with cerebrovascular disease (25% of the population treated), peripheral arterial disease and ischemic cardiac disease (from 5 to 25% of patients with stable cardiovascular disease, and up to 57%).[9,10]

Recently the mechanism of aspirin resistance has been investigated. This term is used to describe the incapacity of the drug to protect patients from thrombotic complications, or to produce an anticipated effect on *in vitro* tests of platelet function. It is not clear whether the effect could be overcome by increasing the dose of the drug, and at least three mechanisms are probably involved in the pathogenesis: enhanced platelet turnover with transient expression of cyclo-oxygenase-2 (COX-2),[11] extra-platelet sources of thromboxane A_2 in patients with acute coronary syndromes[12] and concomitant administration of non-steroidal anti-inflammatory drugs with competition for the common site of action within the cyclo-oxygenase channel.[13]

Pharmacological reperfusion

Aspirin is generally considered to be a weak platelet antagonist, but its therapeutic results are superior to those of far more potent anti-platelet agents with potentially greater clinical effectiveness. ISIS-2 conclusively showed that the administration of aspirin 160 mg/day alone decreased 35-day mortality and reinfarction by 23% in AMI patients and, when combined with streptokinase, decreased short-term mortality and reinfarction by 42%.[14] Aspirin therefore became the standard of care for patients with myocardial infarction. A meta-analysis further demonstrated that aspirin reduced coronary reocclusion and recurrent ischemia after fibrinolysis with streptokinase or alteplase.[15]

In the acute phase of myocardial infarction treated with thrombolytic agents, aspirin has been compared with oral anticoagulants in two trials: the Antithrombotics in the Prevention of Reocclusion In Coronary Thrombolysis (APRICOT) study and the Aspirin/Anticoagulants Following Thrombolysis with Eminase in Recurrent Infarction (AFTER) study.

The endpoint of the APRICOT study was the 3-month reocclusion rate of a patent infarct-related artery demonstrated at angiography up to 48 h after thrombolytic myocardial infarction therapy. Reocclusion occurred in about 30% of the patients, regardless of the use of antithrombotics. There was a reduced rate of reinfarction and revascularization in the aspirin group in comparison with the coumadin or placebo groups.[16] In the AFTER study, the 30-day and 3-month rates of cardiac death and recurrent myocardial infarction were similar in the anti-coagulant and aspirin groups (respectively 11% and 13.2% vs. 11.2% and 12.1%). The trial was stopped early because of its declining enrollment rate.[17]

Mechanical reperfusion

Anti-platelet drugs have not always been evaluated in the setting of primary percutaneous coronary intervention (PCI), but represent a milestone in the prevention of ischemic complications during PCI. Therefore, all information about the use of these drugs during PCI is often empirically applied in the field of emergency percutaneous revascularization. Aspirin should be given promptly to the patient with suspected ST-elevation myocardial infarction, regardless of the strategy of reperfusion.[14]

All initial studies were designed to investigate only the prevention of restenosis after PCI. Although aspirin did not show any benefit on restenosis, the effect on short-term ischemic complications was important.[18] In a study of 376 patients randomly assigned to receive aspirin (990 mg/day) plus dipyridamole (225 mg/day) or placebo, 24 h before angioplasty and continued for 4–7 months, the frequency of peri-procedural myocardial infarction was significantly lower with aspirin plus dipyridamole than with placebo (1.6% vs. 6.9%, $p = 0.011$).[19] In another study, 232 patients were randomized to receive aspirin 325 mg/day or aspirin (same dose) plus dipyridamole 225 mg/day. The rates of peri-procedural myocardial infarction were not significantly different (1.7% vs. 4.3%). Thus the lack of benefit of the addition of dipyridamole to aspirin and the main role of this drug during PCI was demon-strated.[20]

The minimum dosage of aspirin during PCI has not been clearly established, but in an unpublished trial, two dosages of aspirin were evaluated: 80 mg/day versus 1500 mg/day, starting 24 h before balloon angioplasty. No difference was found in the rate of peri-procedural myocardial infarction (3.6% vs. 3.9%) and need for coronary artery bypass graft (CABG) surgery (3.6% vs. 3.7%).[21] The recommen-dation, based on empiric data, is to administer a dose between 75 and 325 mg at least 2 h prior to the procedure.

When aspirin is administered with other anti-platelet agents or anticoagulants, a maximum dose of 162 mg should be used, in order to minimize the risk of bleeding complications. This concept is supported by the observation from the CURE study,[22] where the incidence of major bleeding increased as a function of the aspirin dose, regardless of the association with placebo or clopidogrel in the two arms of the study.

THIENOPYRIDINES

Pharmacokinetics

Ticlopidine and clopidogrel are thienopyridines that selectively inhibit the platelet aggregation induced by ADP. Unlike aspirin, they do not affect the cyclo-oxygenase pathway and arachidonic acid metabolism. Both drugs have short half-lives in the circulation and need hepatic transformation to an active metabolite(s) for their anti-platelet effects. The drugs act by blocking an ADP-binding site on platelets, which inhibits the expression of the glycoprotein IIb/IIIa receptor in the high-affinity configuration that binds fibrinogen and large multimers of vWF.[23] Some evidence suggests that clopidogrel, and probably ticlopidine, may induce an irreversible alteration of the platelet receptor P2Y12, that mediates the inhibition of stimulated adenylyl cyclase activity by ADP, with a selective reduction in the number of ADP-binding sites without changing receptor affinity.[24] This hypothesis can probably explain an abnormal platelet response to ADP associated with mutations of the *P2Y12* gene. The irreversible modification of the ADP receptor can also explain the time-dependent, cumulative inhibition of ADP-induced platelet aggregation obtained with daily dosing, with the onset of action delayed by up to 48–72 h, and slow recovery of platelet function after drug withdrawal (about 1 week).[25]

Platelet inhibition induced by clopidogrel is dose-dependent, with an apparent ceiling effect (40% of inhibition) with a single oral dose of 400 mg, detectable 2 h after the drug administration, and relatively stable up to 48 h. Steady state of action, with inhibition ranging from 50% to 60% is reached after 4–7 days of treatment.[26] The maximum level of platelet inhibition is comparable to that achieved with ticlopidine (500 mg daily), but the latter shows a slower onset of the anti-platelet effect.[27] A much more rapid onset of action can be achieved with a clopidogrel loading dose of 300 mg, rather than the 75-mg dose.[26]

Nevertheless, optimal timing and the size of the loading dose of clopidogrel in the acute clinical setting is still a matter of debate, and doses up to 600 mg are currently administered in patients undergoing percutaneous coronary interventions.

Finally, clopidogrel, like aspirin, shows marked interindividual variability in the inhibitory response based on ADP-induced platelet aggregation, and a variable proportion of patients are currently considered 'non-responders' or resistant to the drug.[28] The mechanism of inter-individual variability is currently under investigation, with two possible hypotheses: a variable metabolic activity of hepatic cytochrome CYP3A4, involved in clopidogrel metabolism, which could modify the systemic bioavailability of the drug, expecially if a concomitant lipophilic drug is administered;[29] and genetic mutations of the *P2Y12* gene, with variation in the rate of affinity between clopidogrel and the platelet receptor.[30]

Both mechanisms and the clinical relevance of clopidogrel resistance need to be further investigated. Currently, no test of platelet function can be routinely recommended to assess the effects of clopidogrel in the individual patient.[31]

Pharmacological reperfusion

Inadequate reperfusion despite thrombolytic therapy occurs in approximately 20% of patients, with a doubled mortality rate. In another 5–8% of patients reocclusion of the infarct-related artery occurs during hospitalization, with triplication of the mortality rate. Arterial thrombi are largely composed of platelets, and are relatively resistant to fibrinolysis, often inducing reocclusion after initial reperfusion. Aspirin alone can reduce the rate of angiographic reocclusion by 22%, but the question of whether the addition of clopidogrel to standard thrombolytic therapy plus aspirin can add further benefit is still under investigation. Clopidogrel has been shown to reduce death and major cardiovascular events in patients with non-ST-elevation acute coronary syndromes,[22,32] and in patients undergoing percutaneous coronary angioplasty.[33,34] The first multicenter trial enrolling 3491 patients with ST-elevation myocardial infarction randomized to standard thrombolytic treatment plus clopidogrel or placebo has recently been published.[35] Patients receiving a fibrinolytic agent, aspirin and heparin were scheduled to undergo coronary angiography 48–192 h after the study drug administration. The primary composite endpoint was the rate of occluded infarct-related artery on angiography (TIMI grade flow 0–1) or death or recurrent myocardial infarction before coronary angiography.

The rates of primary endpoint were 21.7% in the placebo group and 15% in the clopidogrel arm, with an absolute reduction of 6.7 percentage points in the rate and a 36% reduction in the odds of the endpoint in favor of treatment with clopidogrel. Major benefit was driven by the rate of infarct-related artery (reduced from 18.4% to 11.7%, with a 41% reduction in the odds, $p < 0.001$), secondly by the rate of recurrent myocardial infarction (reduced from 3.6% to 2.5%, a 30% reduction in the odds, $p = 0.08$), while no significant effect was evident in the rate of death from any cause (2.2% in the placebo arm and 2.6% in the clopidogrel group, $p = 0.49$). The beneficial effect of clopidogrel was consistent in the prespecified subgroups, on the basis of sex, age, infarct location, type of fibrinolytic agent and heparin used. All angiographic measurements were improved in the clopidogrel group, while no significant effect occurred on the mean degree of ST-segment elevation by 180 min. Clopidogrel therapy was associated with a 21% reduction in the odds of the need of early angiography for clinical indications and urgent revascularization. The rate of a composite endpoint of death, recurrent myocardial infarction and ischemia by 3.5 days was 8.3% in the clopidogrel group and 9.3% in the placebo group (12% odds reduction, $p = 0.27$), while by 30 days the difference was statistically significant (11.6 vs. 14.1%, $p = 0.03$), with odds reduction by 20% with clopidogrel. The significance was mainly driven by the rate of recurrent myocardial infarction (31% reduction with clopidogrel, $p = 0.02$). This trial has demonstrated a clear benefit with the use of clopidogrel in patients with acute myocardial infarction who undergo fibrinolytic therapy, by improving the rates of patency of the infarct-related artery and reducing ischemic complications, but was not sufficiently powered to detect a survival benefit, which was not seen.

Another ongoing trial which is currently exploring the effectiveness of clopidogrel in the acute phase of myocardial infarction is the Clopidogrel and Metoprolol in Myocardial Infarction Trial/Second Chinese Cardiac Study (COMMIT/CCS-2).[36] The mega-trial, designed to assess mortality differences, randomized 46 000 patients with acute myocardial infarction to receive either clopidogrel or placebo within 24 h of symptom onset, with a composite primary endpoint of death, reinfarction or stroke at hospital discharge. The trial has shown a significant risk reduction of the primary endpoint of 9%, with mortality alone reduced by 7%, and reinfarction by 13%. The benefits were not associated with an increased risk of major bleeding or hemorrhagic stroke.[36]

Mechanical reperfusion

It has been shown that the combination of aspirin and thienopyridines has a greater affect on platelet inhibition, due to their complementary mechanism of action.[37] The risk of acute and subacute complications during and after PCI such as subacute vessel closure, which was reported in 3–5% of cases within the first 14 days after stent placement, was strongly reduced with aspirin plus thienopyridines.[38,39]

In the ISAR trial 517 patients who underwent high-risk PCI with Palmaz–Schatz stents (during acute myocardial infarction, with suboptimal results, or with other high-risk clinical or anatomic features) were randomized to receive anti-platelet therapy (aspirin plus ticlopidine) or anticoagulant treatment with aspirin plus heparin and a vitamin K antagonist after stent placement. The composite primary endpoint of cardiovascular death, myocardial infarction, re-surgery for percutaneous transluminal coronary angioplasty (PTCA) or CABG occurred in 1.5% of patients receiving anti-platelet treatment, and in 6.2% of patients treated with anticoagulant therapy, with a rate of subacute stent thrombosis of 0.8% and 5.4%, respectively.[40]

In another important study, the STARS trial,[41] 1653 low-risk patients were randomized to aspirin alone (325 mg/day), aspirin 325 mg plus ticlopidine (500 mg/day) or aspirin 325 mg plus warfarin, after successful stenting. The composite endpoint of death, target lesion revascularization, angiographic thrombosis or myocardial infarction occurred in 3.6% vs. 0.5% vs. 2.7%, respectively ($p < 0.001$). After these two important trials the combination of aspirin and thienopiridines during PCI has become the standard of care.

In two randomized trials clopidogrel has been shown to be safer, easier to administer and at least equally as effective as ticlopidine.[42,43] In a meta-analysis of the CLASSICS[42] trial and of the study of Muller and colleagues,[43] treatment with aspirin plus clopidogrel, compared with aspirin plus ticlopidine after coronary stenting, was associated with a significant reduction in the incidence of major cardiac events (odds ratio 0.50, $p = 0.001$) and mortality (odds ratio 0.43, $p = 0.001$).[44] Greater benefits can be obtained by pretreating patients prior to PCI, as has been shown by the PCI-CURE[33] study and the CREDO trial.[45] In PCI-CURE, treatment of patients with acute coronary syndromes with clopidogrel in the 10 days before PCI resulted in a 30% relative risk reduction of the composite endpoint at 30 days (cardiovascular death, myocardial infarction, urgent target vessel revascularization), while in the CREDO trial a subset of patients pretreated with clopidogrel at least 6 h before elective PCI experienced a 38.6% relative reduction of the combination of death, myocardial infarction and target vessel revascularization; an additional analysis of this study suggested a limitation of the benefit only in patients treated at least 15 h before angioplasty.[34]

This observation has led to further investigation about the delay in the beginning of the platelet inhibitory effect of clopidogrel. It has been shown that a more rapid effect can be achieved by administering a double loading dose of 600 mg instead of 300 mg prior to PCI.[46] This hypothesis has recently been tested in a randomized trial (ARMYDA-2).[47] A total of 255 patients scheduled to undergo PCI were randomized to a loading dose of 600 mg or 300 mg, 4–8 h before the procedure; the primary composite endpoint of death, myocardial infarction and target vessel revascularization at 30 days occurred in 4% of patients pretreated with a 600-mg loading dose versus 12% of patients treated with 300 mg of clopidogrel ($p = 0.041$). The main difference was driven by peri-procedural myocardial infarction, evaluated by a significant CK-MB raise. In the multivariable analysis the high-dose pretreatment was associated with a 50% relative risk reduction of myocardial infarction (odds ratio 0.48, 95% CI 0.15–0.97, $p = 0.044$). Finally, it has been shown that extended treatment with aspirin plus clopidogrel after PCI, either for acute coronary syndromes or elective angioplasty, reduces the rate of ischemic events. In the CREDO trial the 12-month incidence of death, myocardial infarction or stroke was reduced by 26.9% in patients treated with long-term clopidogrel after PCI compared with those receiving aspirin alone. No difference in the rate of minor bleeding complications was found between the two groups, while a slight excess in the rate of major bleeding was found in the clopidogrel arm, mostly related to invasive procedures such as CABG (8.8% vs. 6.7%, $p = 0.07$). In PCI-CURE, major or life-threatening bleeding was similar in the two groups, even when receiving a GP IIb/IIIa inhibitor.

In conclusion, for every patient who undergoes stent placement regardless of during elective or primary angioplasty, aspirin plus thienopyridine treatment is recommended, and clopidogrel over ticlopidine instead of systemic oral anti-coagulation (class 1A). Clopidogrel should be administered with a loading dose of 300 mg at least 6 h before planned PCI (class 1b), and with a loading dose of 600 mg within 6 h before the procedure (class 2C).[48]

GP IIB/IIIA ANTAGONISTS

Pharmacokinetics

GP IIb/IIIa receptor inhibitors block the final pathway of the platelet aggregation induced by any agonist, by inhibiting the binding of fibrinogen to the receptor of activated platelets in a dose-dependent manner. They also have a disaggregating effect on the white thrombus, which becomes a truly thrombolytic effect on platelet aggregates. This 'dethrombotic' effect is related to various mechanisms: the different affinity constants of GP IIb/IIIa inhibitors and fibrinogen for platelet receptors, the reduced platelet release of PAI-1, factor XIII and α_2-antiplasmin, the inhibition of factor XIII and α_2-antiplasmin binding to fibrin, and the inhibition of mechanical clot retraction.[49] GP IIb/IIIa inhibitors remove fibrinogen from the fibrinogen–platelet network because their affinity constant for GP IIb/IIIa receptors is greater than that of fibrinogen. The reduced release of PAI-1 makes the clot more sensitive to fibrinolytic action. As factor XIII and α_2-antiplasmin are important elements in fibrin stabilization, lower concentrations lead to a less organized thrombus that is softer and more easily penetrated by fibrinolytics.

GP IIb/IIIa inhibitors also have anti-proliferative, anti-inflammatory and anticoagulant activity. The fibrinolysis-induced increase in thrombin concentration not only acts as a prothrombotic stimulus, but also reduces fibrinolytic activity by means of the proteolytic activation of TAFI, which inhibits fibrinolysis.

It is possible that, in the presence of potent anti-platelet action, the close correlation between activated platelets and the plasma coagulation phase reduces thrombin generation and finally has an efficacious anticoagulant effect.

The efficacy and safety of the combined use of fibrinolytics and GP IIb/IIIa inhibitors have been assessed in numerous animal studies since 1988. The pathophysiological rationale underlying the use of this combination is based on the presence of platelet thrombi in necrotic arteries after inefficacious fibrinolytic therapy[50] and the disaggregant action of GP IIb/IIIa inhibitors.

Fibrinolytic therapy involves an increase of the prothrombotic state that is related to three mechanisms: the liberation of thrombin from the fibrin–platelet network that in turn involves a catalytic action on the fibrinogen, freeing new thrombin which occurs despite heparin therapy; platelet activation that is mediated directly from fibrinolytic agents or by the increase of thrombin generation; and a liberation of plasmin from plasminogen that makes the activation of factor V – together with Va, Xa and Ca^{++} they make an increase on the platelet surface of thrombin from prothrombin.

In *ex vivo* models, the disaggregant action of GP IIb/IIIa inhibitors has been demonstrated by aggregometric traces showing that the addition of ADP to platelet-rich serum leads to a rapid increase in transmitted light caused by the rapid formation of platelet macroaggregates, and the subsequent addition of abciximab restores the baseline condition of hardly any transmitted light, thus confirming the disaggregation of the macroaggregates.

In studies comparing the efficacy of fibrinolytics alone or in combination with even reduced doses of GP IIb/IIIa inhibitors in animals with experimental myocardial infarction, it has been demonstrated that the combination leads to a more rapid, complete and stable reperfusion than standard fibrinolytic therapy, without any significant increase in hemorrhagic complications.[51,52]

A new finding that has emerged from the studies of combinations of reduced fibrinolytic doses with glycoprotein inhibitors is the high rate of microcirculation restoration and preservation. In addition to improving the patency of the related necrotic artery, the synergistic action of the combined therapy is also shown by the microvessel integrity demonstrated by the rapid normalization of the ST segment.

In TIMI 14, the ST segment normalized in 59% of the patients receiving combined treatment as against 37% of those treated with alteplase alone; among the patients with a TIMI-3 flow, the percentage was also higher in the group that had received alteplase plus abciximab (69% vs. 44%).[53]

There was a direct linear relationship between ST normalization and mortality, which was about 1% in the patients with complete normalization, a little more than 4% in those with 30–70% resolution and about 5% in the non-normalized subjects.

Anti-aggregant and dethrombotic activities transform the platelet-reactive surfaces of complicated plaques into platelet-resistant surfaces, thus leading to a reduction in the distal embolization of platelet aggregates and *'no-reflow'*, and the maintenance of microvascular integrity.

Pharmacological reperfusion

GP IIb/IIIa inhibitors combined with full doses of fibrinolytics

The first pilot clinical study evaluating the use of GP IIb/IIIa inhibitors during fibrinolytic therapy was the Thrombolysis and Angioplasty in Myocardial Infarction study (TAMI-8). This 'safety' study showed that, when administered at scaled doses and at different times (3–15 h after the start of thrombolytic therapy), abciximab did not lead to a greater frequency of hemorrhagic complications when combined with standard tissue-plasminogen activator (t-PA) and heparin doses. Furthermore, there was an increase in the percentage of coronary artery patency at the time of discharge (probably as a result of a reduction in reocclusions) and a low frequency of ischemic events in the patients treated with high doses.[54]

The IMPACT-AMI trial subsequently evaluated the use of different doses of eptifibatide combined with t-PA, aspirin and heparin. The patients treated with high-dose integrilin and standard-dose t-PA showed a higher percentage of reperfusion (TIMI-3 flow), a lower incidence of reocclusion at follow-up angiography and a 43% reduction in the mean time to ST segment normalization in comparison with the control group.[55]

The combination of eptifibatide and streptokinase was tested in a double-blind, placebo-controlled pilot study whose design was similar to that of IMPACT-AMI. There were no significant between-group differences in TIMI-3 flow percentages, but the incidence of hemorrhagic complications was higher in the patients treated with eptifibatide, and the high-dose arm was abandoned because of excess mortality.[56]

The Platelet Aggregation Receptor Antagonist Dose Investigation and reperfusion Gain in Myocardial Infarction (PARADIGM) dose-exploration study evaluated the combination of lamifiban with t-PA or streptokinase in 353 patients. As assessed by means of ST segment monitoring, the frequency, speed and stability of the reperfusion of the necrotic artery were greater in the group treated with t-PA and lamifiban, without any significant increase in hemorrhagic complications.[57]

Cumulative analysis of these studies shows that the combination of fibrinolytics and GP IIb/IIIa inhibitors increases the speed and the percentage of complete reperfusion indicated by angiographic and continuous ST segment monitoring data. However, the study populations were too small and selected (patients at a low risk of stroke) to allow the results to be extrapolated to the general population.

GP IIb/IIIa inhibitors combined with reduced doses of fibrinolytics

The improved reperfusion obtained by combining GP IIb/IIIa inhibitors with low fibrinolytic doses in experimental animal studies, and the risk of hemorrhagic complications when standard fibrinolytic doses are used, led to phase II dose-finding and dose-confirmation clinical trials of combinations including reduced fibrinolytic doses.

Three international randomized phase II dose-finding and confirmation studies have been completed: the Thrombolysis In Myocardial Infarction (TIMI-14) trial, Strategies for Patency Enhancement in the Emergency Department (SPEED) and the INTegrilin and Reduced dose Of thrombolytic in Acute Myocardial Infarction (INTRO-AMI) trial. These, together with the GUSTO V pilot study, have complex designs aimed at identifying the most promising approach for phase III testing.

In TIMI-14, patients with myocardial infarction and ST-segment elevation admitted to hospital within 12 h of symptom onset were treated with aspirin and randomized to one of 14 different pharmacological regimens: full-dose accelerated alteplase, abciximab alone or one of 12 therapeutic regimens combined with different strategies of abciximab and heparin administration (four with scalar doses of streptokinase and eight with scalar doses of alteplase). The primary endpoint was the angiographic evaluation after 90 min; the secondary endpoints were the adverse events occurring during hospitalization and during the course of the 30 days' follow-up. Abciximab combined with reduced doses of alteplase and heparin increased TIMI-3 flow in comparison with a standard fibrinolytic dose. The most efficacious combination was abciximab plus 50 mg of alteplase infused over 60 min, which increased the incidence of a related necrotic artery in comparison with alteplase alone from 43% to 72% after 60 min and from 62% to 77% after 90 min. Combined abciximab and alteplase therapy did not increase the risk of hemorrhage, whereas the combination of abciximab and streptokinase led to an unacceptably high risk.[58] The thrombolytic effect of abciximab was confirmed in the patients receiving abciximab alone, in whom the 32% TIMI-3 flow documented in the related necrotic artery was the same as that obtained with streptokinase in TIMI-1 and GUSTO 1.

The SPEED trial enrolled patients with myocardial infarction and ST-segment elevation within 6 h of the onset of symptoms, and compared treatment with abciximab alone or in combination with five different reteplase regimens (at scalar doses, or as single or double boluses). All of the patients also received aspirin and low-dose heparin. The primary endpoint was the evaluation of TIMI-3 flow in the related necrotic artery after 60 min; the secondary endpoints were the major cardiac events of death or reinfarction, recurrent ischemia requiring revascularization and hemorrhagic complications after 30 days. The therapeutic regimen that guaranteed the greatest percentage of early and complete reperfusion was the combination of abciximab with a double (5 U plus 5 U) reteplase bolus, which led to a 62% TIMI-3 flow after 60 min. The percentage of hemorrhagic complications was similar in the various groups, and similar to the percentages reported in other studies.[59]

The aim of the INTRO-AMI trial was to evaluate the efficacy of different doses of eptifibatide combined with reduced doses of alteplase. The primary endpoint is TIMI-3 flow after 60 min, and the secondary endpoints are ST segment resolution after 180 min and TIMI-3 flow after 90 min. The first phase of the study indicated that the most efficacious treatment for obtaining higher TIMI-3 flow percentages (65% at 60 min and 78% at 90 min) was the combination of various doses of eptifibatide with half the standard dose of rt-PA (a 15-mg bolus followed by a 1-h

35-mg infusion). The dose confirmation phase did not show such impressive patency rates (56% at 60 min and 62% at 90 min) although they were better than those obtained from alteplase alone (40% and 54%, respectively, at 60 and 90 min). The improved patency was associated with a slight increase in bleeding, although this was not statistically significant.

GUSTO V was the first phase III study comparing (in 16 588 patients) the most promising combination of abciximab and reteplase indicated by the SPEED trial (a double bolus of r-PA 5 U plus 5 U and low-dose heparin adjusted on the basis of body weight) with the conventional r-PA double-bolus dose plus standard-dose heparin. Total 30-day mortality (the primary endpoint) was similar in the combination and standard treatment groups (5.6% vs. 5.9%: odds ratio (OR) 0.95; $p = 0.43$), and there was no difference in the incidence of intracranial hemorrhage or non-fatal cerebrovascular accidents. The percentages of almost all of the complications of myocardial infarction, reinfarction, recurrent ischemia and the need for urgent revascularization were significantly lower in the patients receiving the combined therapy, but they also experienced a higher number of hemorrhagic complications and episodes of thrombocytopenia.[60]

The ASSENT (Assessment of the Safety and Efficacy of a New Thrombolytic) 3 trial tested full-dose tenecteplase plus enoxaparin, half-dose tenecteplase with weight-adjusted low-dose unfractionated heparin infusion and abciximab, and standard treatment represented by full-dose tenecteplase with weight-adjusted unfractionated heparin infusion for 48 h. The trial randomized 6095 patients within 6 h of the onset of an acute myocardial infarction to one of three regimens. The combination of reduced-dose tenecteplase and abciximab was associated with similar 30-day mortality compared with full-dose tenecteplase and unfractionated heparin or enoxaparin (6.6% vs. 6.0% vs. 5.4%, respectively, $p = 0.25$). The primary composite endpoints, 30-day mortality, in-hospital reinfarction, or in-hospital refractory ischemia were 11.4% for the enoxaparin group, 11.1% for the abciximab group and 15.4% for the standard treatment group ($p = 0.0001$).

Full-dose TNK with enoxaparin and half-dose lytic plus abciximab and unfractionated heparin both reduced ischemic events compared to standard treatment of full-dose lytic with heparin, but these benefits were obtained at the cost of a higher bleeding rate, particularly in the abciximab group.[61]

The results of these two large-scale trials confirm that the combination of a low dose of fibrinolytic plus glycoprotein inhibitors is an alternative reperfusion strategy, but cannot immediately be applied in the clinical setting, because of the increased risk of hemorrhage, especially in the elderly. Future analyses are necessary (particularly the evaluation of 12-month mortality) in order to define the subgroups of patients in whom the combination has definite advantages over standard treatment.

The ENTIRE-TIMI 23 trial was an open-label, phase 2 angiographic study in which 461 patients were randomized either to full-dose TNK or half-dose TNK plus abciximab, and then further randomized into two corresponding regimens of unfractionated heparin or varying regimens of enoxaparin with and without an initial intravenous bolus. The primary efficacy endpoint was TIMI-3 flow at 60 min that was obtained in each group in approximately 50% of the patients regardless of the lytic regimen used. Patients randomized to combination therapy tended to have higher rates of ST segment resolution at 180 min than those who received standard reperfusion (37% standard, 47% TNK with enoxaparin, 51% associated with unfractionated heparin, 59% associated with enoxaparin). As expected from previous experience, bleeding rates were higher with the combination of half-dose TNK and abciximab, but the use of enoxaparin did reduce bleeding rates, in comparison with the association of half-dose TNK, abciximab and unfractionated heparin.[62]

Mechanical reperfusion

Intravenous GP IIb/IIIa receptor inhibitors have been shown to produce a 35–50% reduction in clinical events in patients with acute coronary syndromes and have been evaluated in patients undergoing primary PCI, but among the three of them (abciximab, eptifibatide, tirofiban) only abciximab has been adequately investigated. Several randomized trials have compared placebo with abciximab during primary angioplasty.[63–66] The RAPPORT showed a reduction of death, reinfarction and urgent target vessel revascularization (TVR) at 30 days, with an excessive bleeding rate.[63] The CADILLAC trial compared routine versus elective stenting in patients undergoing primary PCI, receiving abciximab or placebo. At 30 days the composite primary endpoint of death, reinfarction, revascularization and stroke was higher in the PTCA-alone group, and the lower rates in the other three groups were not significantly affected by the use of abciximab or not.[64] Comparing the primary endpoint in all placebo patients with abciximab patients did not show a statistical difference (18.8% vs. 13.3%). The ADMIRAL trial[65] was the first study to show that abciximab improves clinical outcomes in patients with ST elevation myocardial infarction treated with primary stenting, and the ACE study confirmed these findings, with a reduced incidence of death, reinfarction, TVR, stroke at 30 days (4.5% in the stent plus abciximab vs. 10.5% in the stent-alone group, $p = 0.023$), with the composite primary endpoint reduction mainly driven by the lower rate of reinfarction.[66]

Nevertheless, in the five randomized trials comparing abciximab to placebo, only 1843 in a collective total of 3666 patients actually received abciximab, a relatively small number on which to base recommendations.

In conclusion, ACC/AHA guidelines for the management of patients with ST elevation myocardial infarction state that 'it is reasonable to start treatment with abciximab as early as possible in patients undergoing primary PCI, but given the limitations of the available data set, a class IIa recommendation is assigned'. In a recent meta-analysis all published randomized trials of abciximab in ST elevation myocardial infarction have been examined.[67] Eleven trials involving 27 115 patients were analyzed (12 602 in the abciximab group and 14 513 in the control group), primary endpoints were mortality at 30 days and at long-term follow-up, a secondary endpoint was reinfarction at 30 days and safety endpoints were intracranial bleeding or major bleeding complications as defined by TIMI criteria.

Eight trials were conducted with the use of abciximab during primary angioplasty, and three trials with a full dose of abciximab in addition to a half-dose of fibrinolytic therapy; in one study angioplasty was performed after failed thrombolysis. In all trials except two (ASSENT-3 and ENTIRE-TIMI 23) unfractionated heparin was used.

Abciximab was not associated with a significant reduction in 30-day mortality in all trials combined (5.2% vs. 5.5%, OR 0.97, 95% CI 0.87–1.08; $p = 0.61$) and in fibrinolysis trials (5.8% vs. 5.8%, OR 1.0, 95% CI 0.9–1.12; $p = 0.95$), while a significant reduction was observed only in angioplasty trials (2.4% vs. 3.4%, OR 0.68, 95% CI 0.47–0.99; $p = 0.047$) with a risk reduction of 1% and a number needed to treat of 100 to prevent one death at 30 days' follow-up. A similar result was found for long-term mortality (assessed at 6–12-month follow-up): a significant benefit was observed only in the primary angioplasty trials (4.4% vs. 6.2%, OR 0.69, 95% CI 0.52–0.92, $p = 0.01$), with risk reduction of 1.8% and number needed to treat of 55.6 to prevent one death. For the secondary endpoint (reinfarction at 30 days) a significant reduction with abciximab was observed in all trials combined (2.1 vs. 3.3%, OR 0.63, 95% CI 0.54–0.73; $p < 0.01$), with number needed to treat of 83.3 to prevent one death (111.1 in primary angioplasty, 76.9 in fibrinolysis trials). In all studies combined no intracranial bleeding excess was observed (0.61 vs. 0.62%, OR 1.08, 95% CI 0.79–1.46; $p = 0.62$), with higher incidence of bleeding complications in all trials and in fibrinolysis trials (5.2 vs. 3.1%, OR 1.77, 95% CI 1.55–2.03; $p < 0.01$), whereas no significant difference was observed in angioplasty trials (4.7 vs. 4.1%, OR 1.16, 95% CI 0.85–1.59; $p = 0.36$).

The main finding of this meta-analysis was that adjunctive therapy with abciximab in the setting of ST elevation acute coronary syndrome was associated with a significant reduction in 30 days' recurrence of myocardial infarction regardless of the strategy of reperfusion, with a survival benefit in short- and long-term follow-up observed only in patients undergoing primary angioplasty.

In conjunction with fibrinolytic therapy, a higher risk of major bleeding occurs, with no intracranial bleeding excess except in elderly patients (GUSTO V and ASSENT-3). The benefit observed in the setting of primary angioplasty could be related to the prevention of distal embolization, which is observed in 16% of patients and is associated with impaired myocardial perfusion and higher long-term mortality.

However, benefits on mortality have been shown only in trials enrolling high-risk patients, while low-risk patients are commonly enrolled in the vast majority of trials, with a selection bias that could explain these findings.

The data on tirofiban and eptifibatide are much more limited. However, given the common mode of action, the clinical experience and some angiographic and clinical findings,[68] these drugs have received a class IIb recommendation in the treatment of ST elevation myocardial infarction with primary PCI.

REFERENCES

1. MacIsaac AI, Thomas EJ. Toward the quiescent plaque. J Am Coll Cardiol 1993; 22: 1128–241

2. Falk E, Shah PK, Fuster V. Coronary plaque disruption. Circulation 1995; 92: 657–71

3. Fernandez-Ortiz A, Badimon JJ, Falk E, et al. Characterization of the relative thrombogenicity of atherosclerotic plaque components: implication for plaque rupture. J Am Coll Cardiol 1994; 23: 1562–9

4. Nurden AT, Bihour C, Macchi L, et al. Platelet activation in thrombotic disorders. Nouv Rev Fr Hematol 1993; 35: 67–71

5. Fleming TG. Von Willebrand factor: its function and its measurement in the laboratory. Br J Biomed Sci 1995; 52: 50–7

6. Shah PK. Pathophysiology of plaque rupture and the concept of plaque stabilization. Cardiol Clin 1996; 14: 17–29

7. Ofosu FA, Sie P, Modi GJ, et al. The inhibition of thrombin-dependent positive feedback reaction is critical to the expression of the anticoagulant effect of heparin. Biochem J 1987; 243: 579

8. Shah PK. New insights into the pathogenesis and prevention of acute coronary syndromes. Am J Cardiol 1997; 79: 17–23

9. Gum PA, Kottke-Marchant K, Poggio ED, et al. Profile and prevalence of aspirin resistance in patients with cardiovascular disease. Am J Cardiol 2001; 88: 230–5

10. Sane DC, McKee SA, Malinin AI, et al. Frequency of aspirin resistance in patients with congestive heart failure treated with antecedent aspirin. Am J Cardiol 2002; 90: 893–5

11. Rocca B, Secchiero P, Ciabattoni G, et al. Cyclooxygenase-2 expression is induced during human megakaryopoiesis and characterizes newly formed platelets. Proc Natl Acad Sci USA 2002; 99: 7634–9

12. Cipollone F, Ciabattoni G, Patrignani P, et al. Oxidant stress and aspirin-insensitive thromboxane biosynthesis in severe unstable angina. Circulation 2000; 102: 1007–13

13. Catella-Lawson F, Reilly MP, Kapoor SC, et al. Cyclooxygenase inhibitors and the antiplatelets effects of aspirin. N Engl J Med 2001; 345: 1809–17

14. Randomised trial of intravenous streptokinase, oral aspirin, both, or neither among 17,187 cases of suspected acute myocardial infarction: ISIS-2. ISIS-2 (Second International Study of Infarct Survival) Collaborative Group. Lancet 1988; 2: 349–60

15. Roux S, Christeller S, Ludin E. Effects of aspirin on coronary reocclusion and recurrent ischemia after thrombolysis: a meta-analysis. J Am Coll Cardiol 1992; 19: 671–7

16. Veen G, Meyer A, Verheugt FW, et al. Culprit lesion morphology and stenosis severity in the prediction of reocclusion after coronary thrombolysis: angiographic results of the APRICOT study. Antithrombotics in the Prevention of Reocclusion in Coronary Thrombolysis. J Am Coll Cardiol 1993; 22: 1755–62

17. Julian DG, Chamberlain DA, Pocock SJ, et al. A comparison of aspirin and anticoagulation following thrombolysis for myocardial infarction (the AFTER study): a multicentre unblinded randomised clinical trial. Br Med J 1996; 313: 1429–31

18. Schwartz L, Bourassa M, Lesperance J, et al. Aspirin and dipyridamole in the prevention of restenosis after percutaneous transluminal coronary angioplasty. N Engl J Med 1988; 318: 1714–19

19. Barnathan E, Schwartz J, Taylor L, et al. Aspirin and dipyridamole in the prevention of acute coronary thrombosis complicating coronary angioplasty. Circulation 1987; 76: 125–34

20. Lembo N, Black A, Roubin G, et al. Effect of pretreatment with aspirin versus aspirin plus dipyridamole on frequency and type of acute complications of percutaneous transluminal coronary angioplasty. Am J Cardiol 1990; 65: 422–6

21. Mufson L, Black A, Roubin G, et al. A randomized trial of aspirin in PTCA: effect of high versus low dose aspirin on major complications and restenosis [abstract]. J Am Coll Cardiol 1988; 11: 236A

22. Peters R, Mehta S, Fox K, et al. Effect of aspirin dose when used alone or in combination with clopidogrel in patients with acute coronary syndromes: observations from the Clopidogrel in Unstable angina to prevent Recurrent Events (CURE) study. Circulation 2003; 108: 1682–7

23. Sharis PJ, Cannon CP, Loscalzo J. The antiplatelet effects of ticlopidine and clopidogrel. Ann Intern Med 1998; 129: 394–405

24. Hollopeter G, Jantzen IIM, Vincent D, et al. Identification of the platelet ADP receptor targeted by antithrombotic drugs. Nature 2001; 409: 202–7

25. Herbert JM, Frehel D, Vallee E, et al. Clopidogrel, a novel antiplatelet and antithrombotic agent. Cardiovasc Drug Rev 1993; 11: 180–98

26. Savcic M, Hauert J, Bachmann F, et al. Clopidogrel loading dose regimens: kinetic profile of pharmacodynamics response in healthy subjects. Semin Thromb Haemost 1999; 25: 15–19

27. The CLASSICS Study: Clopidogrel+ASA vs. ticlopidin+ASA in patients with stents. Internist (Berl) 1999; 40 (5 Suppl Clopidogrel): 1–4

28. Gurbel PA, Bliden KP, Hiatt BL, et al. Clopidogrel for coronary stenting: response variability, drug resistance, and the effect of pre-treatment on platelet reactivity. Circulation 2003; 107: 2908–13

29. Lau WC, Waskell LA, Watkins PB, et al. Atorvastatin reduces the ability of clopidogrel to inhibit platelet aggregation: a new drug–drug interaction. Circulation 2003; 107: 32–7

30. Fontana P, Dupont A, Gandrille S, et al. Adenosine diphosphate-induced platelet aggregation is associated with P2Y12 gene sequence variations in healthy subjects. Circulation 2003; 108: 989–95

31. Patrono C, Coller B, Fitzgerald GA, et al. The seventh ACCP conference on antithrombotic and thrombolytic therapy. Platelet-active drugs: the relationships among dose, effectiveness and side effects. Chest 2004; 126: 234S–64S

32. CAPRIE Steering Committee. A randomised, blinded, trial of clopidogrel versus aspirin in patients at risk of ischaemic events (CAPRIE). Lancet 1996; 348: 1329–39

33. Mehta S, Yusuf S, Peters R, et al. Effects of pretreatment with clopidogrel and aspirin followed by long-term therapy in patients undergoing percutaneous coronary intervention: the PCI-CURE study. Lancet 2001; 358: 527–33

34. Steinhubl S, Darrah S, Brennan D, et al. Optimal duration of pretreatment with clopidogrel prior to PCI: data from the CREDO trial. Circulation 2003; 108 (Suppl IV): 374 (abstract)

35. Sabatine MS, Cannon CP, Gibson CM, et al., for the CLARITY-TIMI 28 Investigators. Addition of clopidogrel to aspirin and fibrinolytic therapy for myocardial infarction with ST-segment elevation. N Engl J Med 2005; 352: 1179–89

36. Second Chinese Cardiac Study Collaborative Group. Second Chinese Cardiac Study (COMMIT/CCS-2): a randomized trial of clopidogrel plus aspirin, and of metoprolol, among patients with suspected acute myocardial infarction. Presented at ACC Scientific Sessions, Orlando, FL, 2005

37. Herbert J, Dol F, Bernat A, et al. The antiaggregating and antithrombotic activity of clopidogrel is potentiated by aspirin in several experimental models in the rabbit. Thromb Haemost 1998; 80: 512–18

38. Fischman DL, Leon MB, Baim DS, et al. A randomized comparison of coronary-stent placement and balloon angioplasty in the treatment of coronary artery disease. Stent Restenosis Study Investigators. N Engl J Med 1994; 331: 496–501

39. Serruys P, de Jaegere P, Kiemeneij F, et al. A comparison of balloon expandable stent implantation with balloon angioplasty in patients with coronary artery disease. N Engl J Med 1994; 8: 489–95

40. Schomig A, Neumann FJ, Castrati A, et al. A randomized comparison of antiplatelet and anticoagulant therapy after the placement of coronary artery stents. N Engl J Med 1996; 334: 1084–9

41. Leon M, Baim D, Popma J, et al. A clinical trial comparing three anti-thrombotic regimens after coronary artery stenting. Stent Anticoagulation Restenosis Study Investigators. N Engl J Med 1998; 339: 1665–71

42. Bertrand M, Rupprecht II, Urban P, et al. Double-blind study of the safety of clopidogrel with and without a loading dose in combination with aspirin compared with ticlopidine in combination with aspirin after coronary stenting: the CLopidogrel ASpirin Stent International Cooperative Study (CLASSICS). Circulation 2000; 102: 624–9

43. Muller C, Buttner II, Petersen J, et al. A randomized comparison of clopidogrel and aspirin versus ticlopidine and aspirin after the placement of coronary artery stents. Circulation 2000; 101: 590–3

44. Bhatt D, Marso S, Ilrisch A, et al. Amplified benefit of clopidogrel versus aspirin in patients with diabetes mellitus. Am J Cardiol 2002; 90: 625–8

45. Steinhubl S, Berger P, Mann J, et al. Early and sustained dual oral antiplatelet therapy following percutaneous coronary intervention: a randomized controlled trial. J Am Med Assoc 2002; 288: 2411–20

46. Seyfarth II, Koksch M, Roethig G, et al. Effect of 300- and 450-mg clopidogrel loading doses on membrane and soluble P-selectin in patients undergoing coronary stent implantation. Am Heart J 2002; 143: 118–23

47. Patti G, Colonna G, Pasceri V, et al. Randomized trial of high loading dose of clopidogrel for reduction of periprocedural myocardial infarction in patients undergoing coronary intervention. Results from the ARMYDA-2 trial (Antiplatelet therapy for Reduction of Myocardial Damage during Angioplasty). Circulation 2005; 111: 2099–106

48. Popma JJ, Berger P, Magnus Ohman E, et al. Antithrombotic therapy during percutaneous coronary intervention. The seventh ACCP Conference on antithrombotic and thrombolytic therapy. Chest 2004; 126: 576S–599S

49. Coller BS. Augmentation of thrombolysis with antiplatelet drugs. Overview. Coronary Artery Dis 1995; 6: 911–14

50. Falk E. Thrombosis in unstable angina: pathologic aspects. Cardiovasc Clin 1987; 18: 137–49

51. Yasuda T, Gold HK, Leinbach RC, et al. Lysis of plasminogen activator-resistant platelet-rich coronary artery thrombus with combined bolus injection of recombinant tissue-type plasminogen activator and antiplatelet GPIIb/IIIa antibody. J Am Coll Cardiol 1990; 16: 1728–35

52. Mickelson JK, Simpson PJ, Cronin M, et al. Antiplatelet antibody [7E3 F(ab')2] prevents rethrombosis after recombinant tissue-type plasminogen activator-induced coronary artery thrombolysis in a canine model. Circulation 1990; 81: 617–27

53. de Lemos JA, Antman EM, Gibson M, et al. Abciximab improves both epicardial flow and myocardial reperfusion in ST-elevation myocardial infarction. Observations from the TIMI 14 trial. Circulation 2000; 101: 239–43

54. Kleiman NS, Ohamn EM, Califf RM, et al. Profound inhibition of platelet aggregation with monoclonal antibody 7E3 Fab after thrombolytic therapy: results of the Thrombolysis and Angioplasty in Myocardial Infarction (TAMI) 8 pilot study. J Am Coll Cardiol 1993; 22: 381–9

55. Ohman EM, Leiman NS, Gacioch G, et al. For the IMPACT-AMI Investigators. Combined accelerated tissue-plasminogen activator and platelet glycoprotein IIb/IIIa integrin receptor blockade with integrilin in acute myocardial infarction. Circulation 1997; 95: 846–54

56. Ronner E, van Kesteren HAM, Zijnen P, et al. Combined therapy with streptokinase and integrilin. J Am Coll Cardiol 1998; 31: 191A (abstr.)

57. The PARADIGM Investigators. Combining thrombolysis with the platelet glycoprotein IIb/IIIa inhibitor lamifiban: results of the Platelet Aggregation Receptor Antagonist Dose Investigation and reperfusion Gain in Myocardial Infarction (PARADIGM) trial. J Am Coll Cardiol 1998; 32: 2003–10

58. Antman EM, Giugliano RP, Gibson CM, et al., for the Thrombolysis in Myocardial Infarction (TIMI) 14 Investigators. Abciximab facilitates the rate and extent of thrombolysis: results of Thrombolysis in Myocardial Infarction (TIMI) 14 trial. Circulation 1999; 99: 2720–32

59. Trial of abciximab with and without low-dose reteplase for acute myocardial infarction. Strategies for Patency Enhancement in the Emergency Department (SPEED) Group. Circulation 2000; 101: 2788–94

60. The GUSTO V Investigators. Reperfusion therapy for acute myocardial infarction with fibrinolytic therapy or combination reduced fibrinolytic therapy and platelet glycoprotein IIb/IIIa inhibition: the GUSTO V randomised trial. Lancet 2001; 357: 1905–14

61. The Assessment of the Safety and Efficacy of a New Thrombolytic Regimen (ASSENT)-3 Investigators. Efficacy and safety of tenecteplase in combination with enoxaparin, abciximab, or unfractionated heparin: the ASSENT-3 randomised trial in acute myocardial infarction. Lancet 2001; 358: 605–13

62. Antman EM, Louwerenburg HW, Baars HF, et al., for the ENTIRE-Thrombolysis in Myocardial Infarction (TIMI) 23 Investigators. Enoxaparin as adjunctive antithrombin therapy for ST-elevation myocardial infarction. Results of the ENTIRE-TIMI 23 trial. Circulation 2002; 105: 1642–9

63. Brener SJ, Barr LA, Burchenal JE, et al. Randomized placebo-controlled trial of platelet glycoprotein IIb/IIIa blockade with primary angioplasty for acute myocardial infarction. Reo PRO and Primary PTCA Organization and Randomized Trial (RAPPORT) Investigators. Circulation 1998; 98: 734–41

64. Stone GW, Grines CL, Cox DA, et al., for the CADILLAC Investigators. Comparison of angioplasty with stenting, with or without abciximab, in acute myocardial infarction. N Engl J Med 2002; 346: 957–66

65. Montalescot G, Barragan P, Wittenberg O, et al., for the ADMIRAL Investigators. Platelet glycoprotein IIb/IIIa inhibition with coronary stenting for acute myocardial infarction. N Engl J Med 2001; 344: 1895–903

66. Antoniucci D, Rodriguez A, Hempel A, et al. A randomized trial comparing primary infarct artery stenting with or without abciximab in acute myocardial infarction. J Am Coll Cardiol 2003; 42: 1879–85

67. De Luca G, Suryapranata H, Stone GW, et al. Abciximab as adjunctive therapy to reperfusion in acute ST-segment elevation myocardial infarction. A meta-analysis of randomized trials. J Am Med Assoc 2005; 293: 1759–65

68. Kaul U, Gupta R, Haridas K, et al. Platelet glycoprotein IIb/IIIa inhibition using eptifibatide with primary coronary stenting for acute myocardial infarction: a 30 days follow up study. Catheter Cardiovasc Interv 2002; 57: 497–503

6

Anticoagulants as adjunctive treatment in reperfusion therapy for acute myocardial infarction

Hendrik-Jan Dieker, Freek W A Verheugt

Fibrinolytic therapy has become the standard in most cases of acute ST segment elevation coronary syndromes, since in the 19th and 20th centuries it has become clear that this syndrome is mainly caused by acute thrombotic occlusion of a major epicardial coronary artery. Fibrinolytic therapy is easy to administer in most institutions where patients with acute ST elevation coronary syndromes are presented. The costs are moderate and the benefit is huge, especially with very early and, preferably, prehospital treatment. The outcome of patients treated with fibrinolysis can be improved by adjuvant antiplatelet therapy such as aspirin and, very likely, also by anticoagulant treatment.

The alternative to fibrinolysis as the primary reperfusion strategy in acute ST segment elevation coronary syndromes is primary angioplasty of the infarct-related artery. Although this therapy is superior in the early opening of occluded coronary arteries and in improving early and late survival,[1] it has the main shortcoming of limited availability and, therefore, the need for patient transfer, resulting in long delays. During this delay antithrombotic therapies such as fibrinolytic strategies, advanced anti-platelet or anticoagulation therapy may be of additional value.

Current anticoagulant therapy can be divided into parenteral and oral treatment. Parenteral therapy is aimed at the inhibition of activity and/or generation of thrombin, and oral treatment mainly at inhibition of the formation of coagulation factors involved in the generation and propagation of coronary thrombosis.

ANTI-THROMBIN THERAPY IN FIBRINOLYSIS

Since fibrinolytic therapy is accompanied by intensive thrombin generation and activation, immediate and continuous adjunctive therapy with intravenous unfractionated heparin is recommended.[2] The effect of heparin is mediated through activation of anti-thrombin III, so-called indirect thrombin inhibition. Heparin is thought to block the thrombin activity observed in acute coronary thrombosis and to counteract thrombin release due to clot lysis induced by the fibrinolytic treatment. The paradoxical procoagulant state induced by fibrinolytic therapy is considered to be one of the mechanisms in the occurrence of early coronary reocclusion.[3] However,

97

a benefit of immediate, concomitant heparinization on early patency and reocclusion after fibrinolytic therapy has never been firmly established in patients treated with aspirin.[2,3] As far as the subsequent 48-h infusion is concerned, observational data suggest an effect on recurrent ischemia and clinical reinfarction; a clustering of recurrent ischemic events has been reported early after discontinuation of anti-coagulation therapy.[4]

Both for safety and for efficacy, heparin therapy needs frequent monitoring using activated partial thromboplastin time (aPTT). The level of aPTT at 12 h after lytic therapy has been shown to predict the risk of moderate and severe hemorrhage, and, most importantly, the risk of intracranial bleeding.[2,4] It is noteworthy that patient-related factors have the strongest relationship with bleeding: age, female sex, hypertension and low body weight.[5] Lowering the dose of heparin results in reduction of intracranial hemorrhage without loss of clinical efficacy.[6] In the current guidelines the recommended dose has therefore been changed into a bolus of 60 U/kg to a maximum of 4000 U followed by a continuous infusion for at least 48 h with a target aPTT of 50–70 seconds. Earlier and more frequent monitoring – 3, 6, 12 and 24 h after the first dose[7] – constitutes an additional adjustment.

As an alternative, direct thrombin inhibition has been studied extensively in patients undergoing fibrinolytic therapy for acute infarction. In contrast to indirect thrombin inhibition, direct thrombin inhibitors are also able to inhibit clot-bound thrombin. Moreover, frequent monitoring is not required. In two large clinical trials including over 7000 patients with ST elevation myocardial infarction, hirudin showed no benefit on mortality and a trend towards lower reinfarction rates as compared to heparin. This was at the expense of increased bleeding.[8,9] The same has been observed recently in a trial involving 12 000 patients with the less expensive spe-cific thrombin inhibitor hirulog.[10] Considering the comparable efficacy of these drugs, direct thrombin inhibitors can be used as an alternative to unfractionated heparin, for example in patients with heparin-induced thrombocytopenia.

Low molecular weight heparins have a better bioavailability and induce less platelet activation, and administration can more easily be extended than for unfractionated heparin as a result of the subcutaneous administration. In addition to inhibition of thrombin activity, it has a marked impact higher in the coagulation cascade exerted on factor Xa. Three angiographic trials were performed addressing their impact in conjunction with fibrinolytic therapy. In the placebo-controlled AMI-SK study low molecular weight heparin proved effective with respect to early ST resolution and 5-day patency. In conjunction with t-PA there seemed at least equivalence to unfractionated heparin[11–13] (Table 6.1). In these studies the low molecular weight heparin was given as a bolus together with the lytic drug, and continued subcutaneously twice daily until coronary angiographic evaluation.

Interestingly, in the ASSENT-PLUS trial dalteparin reduced reocclusion and reinfarction during treatment, whereas 30-day reinfarction rates were similar to those of patients in the control arm.[11] A subsidiary analysis in HART-2, studying the subset of patients with TIMI 3 flow at 90-min angiography, suggested lower reocclusion rates at 5–7 days: 9% with unfractionated heparin compared to 3% with enoxaparin ($p = 0.12$).[12] Similar observations have been reported in the PENTAL-

Table 6.1 New anticoagulants as adjuvants to fibrinolytic therapy for acute myocardial infarction

Study	Fibrinolytic agent	New anticoagulant	TIMI flow grade 3	
			New treatment	Unfractionated heparin
			90 minutes	90 minutes
HART-2[12]	rt-PA	Enoxaparin	101/191 (53%)	90/189 (48%)
PENTALYSE[14]	rt-PA	Fondaparinux	148/232 (64%)	57/84 (68%)
			3–5 days	
AMI-SK[13]	SK	Enoxaparin	178/253 (70%)	141/243 (58%)*
ASSENT-PLUS[11]	rt-PA	Dalteparin	140/202 (69%)	110/176 (63%)

*Placebo; $p = 0.01$, numbers are estimates based on the percentages provided in 389 patients with evaluable angiograms
rt-PA, recombinant tissue plasminogen activator; SK, streptokinase

YSE trial, testing pentasaccharide, a specific Xa inhibitor (Table 6.1).[14] In contrast to HART-2, the new antithrombotic regimen was administered longer (5–7 days) than unfractionated heparin (2–3 days). In the subset of patients without signs of recurrent ischemia, reocclusion was reduced from 7% on unfractionated heparin to 0.9% on the pentasaccharide ($p = 0.06$).

The largest randomized trial ever conducted on low molecular weight heparin was the CREATE trial.[15] Subcutaneous reviparin for 7 days was compared to placebo in 15 500 patients from China and India with ST segment elevation myocardial infarction. Placebo was used as comparator, as the clinical impact of adjuvant heparin has never been firmly established. In this trial, 75% of patients were treated with predominantly non-specific fibrinolytic therapy. Interestingly, this was the first clinical trial to demonstrate a mortality benefit of early adjuvant heparin in conjunction with aspirin. At 7 days mortality (8.0 and 8.9%, respectively) and the rate of reinfarction (1.6 and 2.1%, respectively) were significantly reduced and these benefits persisted at 30 days. The total incidence of cerebral bleeding was low, but 2.2 times more frequent with reviparin (Table 6.2).

Two clinical trials have been performed to provide better insight into the safety and efficacy of low molecular weight heparin as compared to unfractionated heparin in combination with fibrin-specific thrombolysis. In the large ASSENT-3 trial enoxaparin (i.v. bolus followed by subcutaneous injections twice daily until discharge) has been compared to unfractionated heparin (bolus followed by infusion for at least 48 h) as adjunct to the bolus lytic agent TNK-tPA (tenecteplase) in over 4000 patients.[16] The enoxaparin regimen turned out to be superior to unfractionated heparin on the combined primary endpoint of 30-day mortality, in-hospital reinfarction and re-ischemia. This benefit was primarily driven by a reduction in recurrent ischemic events, and was lost at 1-year follow-up, which included reinfarctions after hospital discharge.[17] The early clinical benefit was obtained at the expense of a 40% increase in severe, but not cerebral, bleeding. However, in the ASSENT-3 PLUS study cerebral bleeding was unacceptably increased by a regimen including a bolus enoxaparin[18] (Table 6.2). In this randomized trial, 1639 patients treated with prehospitally administered tenecteplase were randomized to a bolus of unfractionated heparin (followed by in-hospital infusion for at least 48 h) or a bolus of enoxaparin (followed by in-hospital subcutaneous injections twice daily). Again, the (longer) administration of enoxaparin resulted in lower rates of recurrent ischemic events. More importantly, however, 12 of the 61 deaths observed on enoxaparin were bleeding-related as compared to only three out of 49 in the control arm.[18]

Thus, current anti-thrombin therapy after fibrinolytic therapy seems to be optimal with unfractionated heparin, which is given as a bolus together with the lytic (preferably tenecteplase) and continued for at least 48 h. An alternative after the bolus unfractionated heparin could be enoxaparin or reviparin subcutaneously until hospital discharge. This, in view of the previously described observations that longer-term administration of anti-thrombin therapy might reduce in-hospital reocclusion and recurrent ischemic events. These recommendations originate from several randomized angiographic observations and three large clinical trials. Definite guidelines should be founded on more clinical data, especially those with

Table 6.2 Risks of using novel anticoagulant therapy as an adjuvant to fibrinolytic therapy for acute myocardial infarction

Study	Fibrinolytic agent	New anticoagulant	Cerebral bleeding		
			New anticoagulant	Placebo	
					Unfractionated heparin
CREATE[15]	any*	Reviparin	22/7780 (0.3%)	** 10/7790 (0.1%)	
PENTALYSE[14]	rt-PA	Fondaparinux	1/241 (0.4%)	0/85 (0.0%)	
ASSENT-3[16]	TNK-tPA	Enoxaparin	18/2040 (0.9%)		19/2038 (0.9%)
ASSENT-3 PLUS[18]	TNK-tPA	Enoxaparin	18/818 (2.2%)		*** 8/821 (1.0%)
Total			36/2858 (1.3%)		**** 27/2859 (0.9%)

*Only 75% fibrinolysis (mainly non-fibrin specific); **$p = 0.03$; ***$p = 0.05$; ****$p = 0.18$

regard to safety. This issue is currently studied in the EXTRACT-TIMI 25 clinical mega-trial, in which age-dependent doses of subcutaneous injections of enoxaparin with or without bolus will be compared to unfractionated heparin bolus plus infusion after lytic therapy with either alteplase, tenecteplase, reteplase or strepto-kinase. The role of the pentasaccharide fondaparinux in reperfusion therapy, either fibrinolysis or primary angioplasty, is currently being evaluated in the large OASIS-6 trial.

ANTI-THROMBIN THERAPY IN PRIMARY ANGIOPLASTY

The role of anti-thrombin therapy in primary angioplasty for ST elevation acute coronary syndromes has not been studied in large trials. It is generally given in order to prevent thrombus formation at the site of the ruptured plaque, at iatrogenic vessel injury and on the indwelling catheter. Guidelines recommend an intravenous bolus of unfractionated heparin either to an activated clotting time (ACT) between 250 and 350 seconds or in a weight-adjusted manner (usually 100 IU/kg).[19] Heparin bolus as adjunct to glycoprotein IIb/IIIa antagonists for this indication needs a lower dose with an ACT between 200 and 250 seconds or weight adjusted at 50–60 IU/kg (see Chapter 5). Heparin infusion is usually given for at least 48 h as part of the standard therapy for acute myocardial infarction. To minimize the risk of puncture-site bleeding, special care should be taken with regard to the removal of the vascular sheath, especially when heparin infusion is given. In case of glycoprotein IIb/IIIa antagonist use, early sheath removal at an ACT of < 175 seconds and the use of a reduced bolus of heparin without additional infusion seems to lower the risk of bleeding.[20]

High-dose bolus of heparin (up to 300 U/kg) has been studied in the facilitation of primary angioplasty and has not been found to be helpful.[21] A high-dose bolus of heparin given in the referring hospital, ambulance or emergency room of the angioplasty center was only associated with a higher patency rate pre-angioplasty in patients with symptoms of less than 2 h.[21] A bolus of heparin (5000 U) in combination with aspirin during transferral for primary angioplasty is associated with a higher pre-intervention patency rate as compared to no heparin or aspirin.[22] There have been no reports on a specific benefit for the use of low molecular weight heparins as an adjunct for primary angioplasty for ST elevation myocardial infarction.[19] In the primary angioplasty arm of GUSTO-IIb consisting of 503 patients, direct thrombin inhibition with hirudin showed a trend towards less mortality in comparison with heparin (4.7% vs. 6.1%, respectively), but no differences in reinfarction.[23]

ORAL ANTICOAGULATION AFTER MYOCARDIAL INFARCTION

Given the promising observations of a prolonged in-hospital regimen of both anti-platelet and anti-thrombin therapy, oral anticoagulation seems a logical follow-up therapy after discontinuation of heparin in thrombotic disorders. The impact of oral anticoagulation (Tables 6.3 to 6.5) is effected through interference with the production of vitamin K-dependent coagulation factors (II, VII, IX, X).[24]

As a single antithrombotic regimen after myocardial infarction, it has been tested extensively in the past three decades.[24] Not until recently, however, has the combination of oral anticoagulation with the standard anti-platelet regimen after myocardial infarction (aspirin) been evaluated. This combination has become more appealing since the introduction of lower doses of aspirin (maximum 325 mg daily), and the improved safety of oral anticoagulation after the introduction of the international normalized ratio (INR).

The first trial to demonstrate the efficacy of oral anticoagulation on top of aspirin was the small ATACS study,[25] in which 214 patients with unstable angina pectoris or non-ST elevation myocardial infarction were randomized to aspirin alone or to aspirin plus heparin followed by dose-adjusted warfarin with a mean INR of 2.3. Despite the promising results of this small trial, several large-scale trials have been performed in which no benefit of this combined regimen was demonstrated. In the CARS trial[26] over 9000 patients early after myocardial infarction were randomized to aspirin alone (daily dose 160 mg), or to aspirin (80 mg daily) combined with a fixed dose of warfarin (1 or 3 mg daily; reached INRs 1.1 and 1.5, respectively). After 1.2 years no differences were observed in death and recurrent myocardial infarction. More or less the same disappointing results were seen after 2.5 years in the over 5000 patients CHAMP study,[27] with a reached INR of 1.8. In that trial patients were randomized to aspirin alone 160 mg daily or to aspirin 80 mg daily plus warfarin, which was laboratory monitored to an INR of 1.5 to 2.5. Finally, the most recent trial is the Swedish LOWASA study, which evaluated combined fixed low-dose oral anticoagulation (1.25 mg daily) and antiplatelet therapy (aspirin 75 mg daily) in comparison to aspirin (75 mg daily) alone in 3300 post-myocardial infarction patients. This regimen, where INR data are lacking, did not show a clinical benefit of the combined treatment, whereas severe bleeding was increased.[28]

The APRICOT-2 angiographic follow-up study[29] investigated the role of combined anticoagulant (median INR 2.6)/anti-platelet therapy versus aspirin alone (80 mg daily) in over 300 patients with a patent infarct artery after fibrinolytic therapy. To date, this is the only trial studying this combined antithrombotic regimen specifically in patients treated with fibrinolysis. The combined treatment reduced angiographic reocclusion at 3 months from 28% with aspirin to 15% ($p < 0.02$). The secondary endpoints, recurrent infarction and the need for revascularization, were markedly reduced on the prolonged combined antithrombotic regimen and safety was excellent (no intracranial hemorrhage; only minor bleedings were doubled by coumadin plus aspirin). The clinical ASPECT-2 trial[30] studied full-intensity (mean INR 3.2) coumadin alone (without aspirin), the combination medium-intensity coumadin (mean INR 2.4) and aspirin 80 mg daily, and aspirin 80 mg daily alone in 993 patients randomized within 2 weeks after myocardial infarction. About 50% of the patients had received fibrinolytic therapy in the acute phase. The 1-year death and reinfarction rate of 8% on aspirin alone was reduced by 45% and 50% in the combination and coumadin-alone groups,

Table 6.3 Randomized angiographic studies of oral anticoagulation on top of aspirin as compared to aspirin alone after acute coronary syndromes

Study	Year	n	INR target	INR reached	ASA dose (mg)	% (re)occlusion		RR	p Value	Fup (months)
						ASA+OAC	ASA			
Williams[32]	1997	57	2.0–2.5	2.0	150	4%	33%	n.a.	0.02*	3
APRICOT-2[29]	2002	310	2.0–3.0	2.6	80	15%	28%	0.55 (0.33–0.90)	<0.02	3

*p Value by Fisher exact test; n, number of patients randomized; INR, international normalized ratio; ASA, aspirin; OAC, oral anticoagulation; RR, relative risk; Fup, follow-up period; n.a., not applicable

Table 6.4 Randomized clinical studies of fixed low-dose oral anticoagulation on top of aspirin as compared to aspirin alone after acute coronary syndromes

Study	Year	n	INR target	INR reached	ASA dose (mg)	% mortality, (re)MI, stroke		RR	p Value	Fup (months)
						ASA+OAC	ASA			
CARS[26]	1997	8803	1 mg qd 3 mg qd	1.1 1.5	80 vs. 160	11.6% 8.7%	10.0%	1.18 (1.07–1.31) 0.98 (0.90–1.07)	<0.01 0.26	14 14
LOWASA[28]	2004	3300	1.25 mg qd	n.p.	75	28.1%	28.8%	0.98 (0.91–1.06)	0.67	60

n, number of patients randomized; INR, international normalized ratio; ASA, aspirin; OAC, oral anticoagulation; RR, relative risk; Fup, follow-up period; qd, once daily; n.p., not published

Table 6.5 Randomized clinical studies of oral dose-adjusted anticoagulation on top of aspirin as compared to aspirin alone after acute coronary syndromes

Study	Year	n	INR target	INR reached	ASA dose (mg)	% mortality, (re)MI, stroke ASA+OAC	ASA	RR	p Value	Fup (months)
CHAMP[27]	2002	5059	1.5–2.5	1.9	80 vs. 160	17.6%	17.3%†	1.01 (0.94–1.09)	0.76	33
OASIS-2[33]	2001	3712	2.0–2.5	n.p.	Not specified	7.6%	8.3%	0.90 (0.72–1.14)	0.40	5
good compliers		1821				6.1%	8.9%	0.68 (0.48–0.95)	0.02	
poor compliers		1891				9.0%	7.8%	1.17 (0.86–1.60)	0.33	
ATACS[25]	1994	214	2.0–3.0	2.3	160	12.8%	25.7%	0.62 (0.40–0.97)	0.02	3
ASPECT-2[30]	2002	668	2.0–2.5	2.4	80	5.0%	9.0%	0.52 (0.28–0.98)	< 0.05	12
WARIS-2[31]	2002	2414	2.0–2.5	2.2	75 vs. 160	15.0%	20.0%	0.71 (0.60–0.83)	< 0.01	48
Total		**12 067**				**13.2%**	**14.7%**	**0.89 (0.82–0.98)**	**0.01***	

†Mortality, primary endpoint; *compared using the Mantel–Haenzel method; n, number of patients randomized; INR, international normalized ratio; ASA, aspirin; OAC, oral anticoagulation; RR, relative risk; Fup, follow-up period; qd, once daily; good/poor compliers, oral anticoagulation use in over/less than 70% patients at 35 days; n.p., not published

respectively ($p = 0.05$). Also in this trial bleeding was low (major bleeding for the combination 1.8%, for aspirin alone 0.9%). Despite promising efficacy findings, both trials are too small to be conclusive on safety.

The WARIS-2 trial has been carried out in Norway in 3600 patients, who survived myocardial infarction, and compared aspirin (160 mg daily) alone with either full-intensity oral anticoagulation (target INR 2.8 to 4.2) alone or the combination of low-dose aspirin (75 mg daily) with medium-intensity oral anti-coagulation (target INR 2.0 to 2.5). Over a 4-year follow-up period a 30% reduction in the combined endpoint of death, reinfarction and stroke was observed with medium-intensity warfarin (mean INR 2.2) plus aspirin as compared to aspirin alone, with an acceptable safety profile.[31]

In contrast to the larger clinical trials, in APRICOT-2[29] coumadin was initiated early, within 48 h of fibrinolysis, during heparinization. Parenteral anticoagulation was discontinued when the target INR was reached. Thus, an uninterrupted, prolonged combined antithrombotic regimen was realized. A similar strategy was followed in a smaller angiographic trial performed in a mixed patient population recovering from acute coronary syndromes reporting comparable findings.[32] The only clinical trial with this regimen was OASIS-2, addressing non-ST elevation acute coronary syndromes.[33] Importantly, a stratified comparison on the compliance per center showed that the potential efficacy was largely dependent on the level of compliance.

The positive impact of coumadin on long-term reocclusion and recurrent ischemic events seems to corroborate well with the in-hospital clinical benefit seen with the new prolonged anti-thrombin regimens in the angiographic studies[11–14] and the clinical ASSENT-3 and CREATE trials.[15,16]

A relatively new oral anticoagulant, the direct thrombin blocker ximelagatran, has been tested against placebo in 1888 patients following myocardial infarction treated with aspirin. Death, reinfarction and stroke were significantly reduced by 34% from 11.1% to 7.4% with an acceptable bleeding risk.[34] However, transient unacceptable liver enzyme elevation occurred in this trial and others on atrial fibrillation, which proved the Achilles' heel of the agent.[35]

In conclusion, adding oral anticoagulants to anti-platelet therapy does not show benefit when a fixed low-dose or low-intensity (INR < 2) regimen is used.[36] Adequate dose-adjusted anticoagulation with INRs over 2.0 seems to improve clinical and angiographic results with and probably without fibrinolytic therapy, with an acceptable bleeding risk.

CONCLUSIONS

Anticoagulation therapy seems to be essential to optimize outcome after reperfusion therapy for acute myocardial infarction. Unfractionated heparin is used widely for this purpose, both in fibrinolysis and in primary angioplasty. The more expensive specific thrombin inhibitors such as hirudin and hirulog do not seem to be inferior to unfractionated heparin and can be used in case of heparin-induced thrombocytopenia. So far, the best angiographic and clinical results are obtained with low molecular weight heparin, but its safety is still a matter of debate and, therefore, it cannot be recommended until more studies have been done.

Long-term adequate dose-adjusted coumadin (INR > 2.0) on top of aspirin is effective after fibrinolysis for acute myocardial infarction, when compared to aspirin alone. Important issues are timing and adequacy of the intensity of therapy. Fixed low-dose therapy or dose-adjusted treatment with a reached INR below 2.0 do not lead to better outcomes following myocardial infarction. Bleeding is acceptable since the introduction of lower doses of aspirin.

REFERENCES

1. Keeley EC, Boura JA, Grines CL. Primary coronary angioplasty versus intravenous fibrinolytic therapy for acute myocardial infarction: a quantitative review of 23 randomised trials. Lancet 2003; 361: 13–20

2. Collins R, Peto R, Baigent C, Sleight P. Aspirin, heparin, and fibrinolytic therapy in acute myocardial infarction. N Engl J Med 1997; 336: 847–60

3. Verheugt FWA, Meijer A, Lagrand WK, Van Eenige MJ. Reocclusion, the flipside of coronary thrombolysis. J Am Coll Cardiol 1996; 27: 766–73

4. Granger CB, Hirsh J, Califf RM, et al. Activated partial thromboplastin time and outcome after thrombolytic therapy for acute myocardial infarction: results from the GUSTO-1 trial. Circulation 1996; 93: 870–8

5. Gore JM, Granger CB, Sloan MA, et al. Stroke after thrombolysis: mortality and functional outcome after thrombolytic therapy for acute myocardial infarction: results from the GUSTO trial. Circulation 1995; 92: 2811–18

6. Gugliano RP, McCabe CH, Antman EM, et al. Lower-dose heparin with fibrinolysis is associated with lower rates of intracranial hemorrhage. Am Heart J 2001; 141: 742–50

7. Van de Werf F, Ardissino D, Betriu A, et al. Management of acute myocardial infarction in patients presenting with ST-elevation. Eur Heart J 2003; 24: 28–66

8. GUSTO-IIb Investigators. A comparison of recombinant hirudin with heparin for the treatment of acute coronary syndromes. N Engl J Med 1996; 335: 775–82

9. Antman EM, for the TIMI 9B investigators. Hirudin in acute myocardial infarction. Thrombolysis In Myocardial Infarction (TIMI) 9B trial. Circulation 1994; 90: 1624–30

10. HERO-2 Investigators. Thrombin-specific anticoagulation with bivalirudin versus heparin in patients receiving fibrinolytic therapy for acute myocardial infarction: the HERO-2 trial. Lancet 2001; 358: 1855–63

11. Wallentin L, Bergstrand L, Dellborg DM, et al. Low-molecular-weight heparin (dalteparin) as an adjunct to rt-PA (alteplase) for improvement of coronary artery patency in acute myocardial infarction – the ASSENT PLUS study. Eur Heart J 2003; 24: 897–908

12. Ross AM, Molhoek P, Lundergan C, et al. Randomized comparison of enoxaparin, a low molecular weight heparin, with unfractionated heparin adjunctive to tissue plasminogen activator thrombolysis and aspirin: second trial of Heparin and Aspirin Reperfusion Therapy (HART II). Circulation 2001; 104: 648–52

13. Simoons ML, Alonso A, Krzeminska-Pakula M, et al. Early ST segment elevation resolution: predictor of outcome and angiographic patency in patients with acute myocardial infarction. Results of the AMI-SK study. Eur Heart J 2002; 23: 1282–90

14. Coussement PK, Bassand JP, Convens C, et al. A synthetic factor-Xa inhibitor (ORG13540/SR9017A) as an adjunct to fibrinolysis in acute myocardial infarction. The PENTALYSE-study. Eur Heart J 2001; 22: 1716–24

15. CREATE Trial Group Investigators. Effect of reviparin, a low-molecular-weight heparin, on mortality, reinfarction and strokes in patients with acute myocardial infarction presenting with ST-segment elevation. J Am Med Assoc 2005; 293: 427–36

16. ASSENT-3 Investigators. Efficacy and safety of tenecteplase with enoxaparin, abciximab or unfractionated heparin: the ASSENT-3 randomised trial in acute myocardial infarction. Lancet 2001; 358: 605–13

17. Wallentin L. One year follow-up data of the ASSENT-3 trial. Presented at the 24th Congress of the European Society of Cardiology, 31 August through 4 September 2002, Berlin, Germany

18. Wallentin L, Goldstein P, Amstrong PW, et al. Efficacy and safety of tenecteplase in combination with the low-molecular-weight heparin enoxaparin or unfractionated heparin in the prehospital setting. The ASSENT-3 PLUS randomized trial in acute myocardial infarction. Circulation 2003; 108: 135–42

19. Silber S, Albertsson P, Aviles FF, et al. ESC guidelines for percutaneous coronary interventions. Eur Heart J 2005; 26: 804–47

20. The PROLOG Investigators. Standard versus low-dose weight-adjusted heparin in patients treated with the platelet glycoprotein IIb/IIIa receptor antibody fragment abciximab (c7E3 Fab) during percutaneous coronary revascularization. Am J Cardiol 1997; 79: 286–91

21. Liem AL, Zijlstra F, Ottervanger JP, et al. High dose bolus heparin as pretreatment of primary angioplasty in acute myocardial infarction: the Heparin in Early Patency (HEAP) randomized trial. J Am Coll Cardiol 2000; 35: 600–4

22. Zijlstra F, Ernst N, De Boer MJ, et al. Influence of pre-hospital administration of aspirin and heparin on initial patency of the infarct-related artery in patients with acute ST-elevation myocardial infarction. J Am Coll Cardiol 2002; 39: 1733–7

23. GUSTO-IIb Angioplasty Substudy Investigators. A clinical trial comparing primary coronary angioplasty with tissue plasminogen activator for acute myocardial infarction. N Engl J Med 1997; 336: 1621–8

24. Brouwer MA, Verheugt FWA. Oral anticoagulants in acute coronary syndromes. Circulation 2002; 105: 1270–4

25. Cohen M, Adams PC, Parry G, et al. Combination antithrombotic therapy in unstable rest angina and non-Q-wave infarction in nonprior aspirin users. Primary end-points analysis from the ATACS trial. Circulation 1994; 89: 81–8

26. Coumadin Aspirin Reinfarction Study (CARS) Investigators. Randomised double-blind trial of fixed low-dose warfarin with aspirin after myocardial infarction. Lancet 1997; 350: 389–96

27. Fiore LD, Ezekowitz MD, Brophy MT, et al., for the Combination Hemotherapy and Mortality Prevention (CHAMP) Study Group. Department of veteran affairs cooperative studies program clinical trial comparing combined warfarin and aspirin with aspirin alone in survivors of acute myocardial infarction. Primary results of the CHAMP study. Circulation 2002; 105: 557–63

28. Herlitz J, Holm J, Peterson M, et al. Effect of fixed low-dose warfarin added to aspirin in the long term after acute myocardial infarction. Eur Heart J 2004; 25: 232–9

29. Brouwer MA, Van den Bergh PJPC, Vromans RPJW, et al. Aspirin plus medium intensity coumadin versus aspirin alone in the prevention of reocclusion after successful thrombolysis for suspected acute myocardial infarction: results of the APRICOT-2 study. Circulation 2002; 106: 659–65

30. Van Es RF, Jonker JJC, Verheugt FWA, Deckers JW, Grobbee DE. Aspirin, coumadin or both after acute coronary syndromes: results of the ASPECT-2 trial. Lancet 2002; 360: 109–13

31. Hurlen M, Abdelnoor M, Smith P, Erikssen J, Arnesen H. Warfarin, aspirin, or both after myocardial infarction. N Engl J Med 2002; 347: 969–74

32. Williams MJA, Morison IM, Parker JH, Stewart RH. Progression of the culprit lesion in unstable coronary artery disease with warfarin and aspirin versus aspirin alone: preliminary study. J Am Coll Cardiol 1997; 30: 364–9

33. The Organisation to Assess Strategies for Ischemic Syndromes (OASIS-2) Investigators. Effects of long-term, moderate-intensity oral anticoagulation in addition to aspirin in unstable angina. J Am Coll Cardiol 2001; 37: 475–84

34. Wallentin L, Wilcox R, Weaver W, et al. Oral ximelagatran for secondary prophylaxis after myocardial infarction: the ESTEEM randomised controlled trial. Lancet 2003; 362: 789–97

35. Verheugt FWA. Can we pull the plug for warfarin in atrial fibrillation? Lancet 2003; 362: 1686–7

36. Anand SS, Yusuf S. Oral anticoagulation in patients with coronary artery disease. J Am Coll Cardiol 2003; 41: 62S–9S

7

Pharmacological interventions in reperfusion therapy for acute myocardial infarction

Sanjaya Khanal, W Douglas Weaver

Acute myocardial infarction (AMI) accounts for half of the 15.5 million cardiovascular deaths annually worldwide.[1] The outcome of hospitalized patients with AMI has improved dramatically, owing to advances in detection, monitoring and therapy for this condition.

AMI is usually a result of thrombosis of a ruptured atherosclerotic plaque inside a coronary artery of an affected patient.[2] If the thrombosis results in complete occlusion of the vessel, it usually manifests as ST segment elevation myocardial infarction. On the other hand, if the occlusion is incomplete or temporary, it results in non-ST elevation acute coronary syndrome. Because rapid myocardial necrosis results from cessation of blood flow in the myocardium, it is essential that antegrade flow to the myocardium be restored rapidly and efficiently in patients with ST segment elevation myocardial infarction to prevent continued damage to the left ventricular myocardium. Since the amount of myocardial damage during AMI is directly related to long-term prognosis, myocardial salvage has been the primary goal of treatment of AMI.[3] In the immediate term, the major risk of mortality is from ventricular fibrillation as a result of the myocardial ischemia. Therefore, rapid defibrillation capability in the field or in the hospital results in improved survival in patients with AMI.[4] The other major determinant of prognosis is the ability to restore normal flow in the infarct-related artery expeditiously. This can be achieved by either fibrinolysis or direct percutaneous coronary intervention (PCI). If highly trained operators can carry it out expeditiously, percutaneous coronary intervention results in better outcome in patients with ST segment elevation myocardial infarction. However, a great majority of the patients who present with AMI do not have ready access to PCI and are treated with fibrinolytics initially. This strategy has resulted in significant improvement in outcome compared to placebo in randomized trials.[3,5] Further improvements have been achieved by combining anti-platelet agents such as aspirin and antithrombotic agents with timely administration of fibrinolytics.

Only half of the patients initially treated with fibrinolytics achieve normal blood flow in the infarct-related artery.[6] Except for the patients treated very early in the AMI course, most patients have evidence of significant myocardial damage. In addition to reperfusion, many therapeutic regimens have the potential to limit the myocardial damage, reduce post-AMI complications and improve short- and long-term outcome in these patients. Therefore, in addition to reperfusion therapy, many pharmacological agents have been investigated to treat and improve outcome in patients with AMI.

β-BLOCKERS

β-Blockers have been demonstrated to reduce morbidity and mortality in patients with AMI (Table 7.1). As a class of agents, β-blockers act on cellular β-receptors and block their actions, resulting in various physiological effects in the heart and other tissues. Clinically, they commonly reduce blood pressure and heart rate, but physiologically they reduce myocardial ischemia (MI) by decreasing myocardial oxygen demand during AMI. They also reduce myocardial infarct size, positively modulate the myocardial metabolism, stabilize cellular membranes, reduce reperfusion injury and increase the threshold for cardiac arrhythmia. In the longer term, they help prevent adverse remodeling of the left ventricle, improve myocardial energetics and reduce vulnerability to malignant arrhythmia. Therefore, they have been studied extensively as adjunctive therapy of patients with AMI.

Yusuf et al. demonstrated that early intravenous β-blockade reduced infarct size and arrhythmias in patients treated early with intravenous and continued on oral atenolol.[7] A similar effect was shown with timolol administered during AMI by Hammerman et al.[8] and the International Collaborative Study Group.[9]

Hjalmarson et al. treated 1395 patients with metoprolol or placebo on presentation with AMI and continued for 90 days. The mortality in patients in the metoprolol group was 5.7% compared to 8.9% in the placebo group (p < 0.03).[10]

The Beta-Blocker Heart Attack trial demonstrated reduction in 27-month mortality with administration of propanolol after 5 days of AMI.[11] A similar reduction was demonstrated in the Norwegian study using timolol.[12]

The Metoprolol in Acute Myocardial Infarction (MIAMI) trial demonstrated that early intravenous metoprolol administration resulted in reduced myocardial infarct size within 7 days.[13] The large First International Study of Infarct Survival (ISIS-1), a 16 027 patient trial, randomized AMI patients to receive intravenous

Table 7.1 Randomized trials of β-blockers in acute myocardial infarction

Study	Agent	Patients (n)	Duration	RR of death	p Value
ISIS-1	Atenolol	16 027	7 days	0.85 (0.73–0.99)	< 0.04
MIAMI	Metoprolol	5778	15 days	0.87 (0.67–1.08)	0.29
TIMI-IIB	Metoprolol	1434	6 days	1.00	0.98
Norwegian	Timolol	1884	33 months	0.61 (0.46–0.80)	< 0.001
BHAT	Propanolol	3837	25 months	0.72 (0.64–0.80)	< 0.005
CAPRICORN	Carvedilol	1959	1.3 years	0.77 (0.60–0.98)	0.03

(5–10 mg) followed by oral (100 mg/day) atenolol.[5] There was 15% reduction in mortality within 1 week that persisted to 1 year.

The Thrombolysis in Myocardial Infarction (TIMI)-IIB trial randomized patients to early and late metoprolol (initially 5 mg intravenously three times, 50 mg twice the first day and 100 mg twice daily subsequently) in combination with the fibrinolytic reteplase.[14] Although there was no mortality difference at 1 year, the early β-blocker treatment group had lower mortality and lower reinfarction rates at 6 weeks.

The CAPRICORN study randomized 1959 patients with acute myocardial infarction and left ventricular ejection fraction of ≤ 40% to carvedilol or placebo and demonstrated reduction in all-cause mortality (12% vs. 15%, HR 0.77, $p = 0.031$).[15]

From these clinical trials, it is clear that β-blockers reduce myocardial ischemia, chest pain, infarct size, cardiac arrhythmias, repeat infarctions and short- and long-term mortality in patients with AMI.

Recommendations

Current recommendations for β-blockers in AMI are to use them in all patients without contraindications.[16] Ideally, β-blocker therapy (e.g. 5 mg of metoprolol or atenolol, 2–3 doses over the first 15 min) should be administered intravenously on presentation with AMI. Oral β-blockers should be continued in-hospital and long term to reduce long-term mortality. The only absolute contraindications to β-blockade are cardiogenic shock, significant acute pulmonary edema, severe hypotension, bradycardia and active bronchospastic disease. Adequate doses of β-blockers (≥ 100 mg of metoprolol or equivalent a day) should be administered in all eligible patients long term.

ANGIOTENSIN CONVERTING ENZYME INHIBITORS

Angiotensin converting enzyme (ACE) inhibitors block the enzyme that converts angiotensin I to angiotensin II in the blood and tissues. The renin–angiotensin system has been associated with progression of atherosclerosis, endothelial dysfunction, myocardial hypertrophy and ventricular dysfunction. The hyperactivity of the renin–angiotensin system adds to the up-regulation of the adverse neurohumeral cascade that results in worsening left ventricular dysfunction in patients with myocardial damage. Therefore, blockade of this system with ACE inhibitors results in better outcome in patients with congestive heart failure and asymptomatic left ventricular dysfunction.[17,18] In patients with AMI, the left ventricle adversely remodels leading to dilatation of the chamber and sometimes aneurysm formation.[19] ACE inhibitors effectively prevent adverse remodeling with improved long-term ventricular function.

Multiple randomized studies had been shown to improve prognosis of patients with left ventricular dysfunction with the use of ACE inhibitors.[17,18] Similar benefit has been demonstrated in patients with MI (Table 7.2). The Survival And

Ventricular Enlargement (SAVE) trial was the first conclusive study to demonstrate similar beneficial effects in patients with post-MI left ventricular dysfunction.[20] The study randomized 2231 patients with left ventricular ejection fraction of < 40% to receive either captopril or placebo 3–16 days after their MI. There was 19% relative reduction in mortality and 25% reduction in progression of heart failure in patients taking captopril. The Acute Infarction Ramipril Efficacy (AIRE) study showed similar benefit with the use of ramipril and the Trandolapril Cardiac Evaluation (TRACE) study with trandolapril.[21,22] The Survival of Myocardial Infarction Long-term Evaluation (SMILE) study demonstrated 25% reduction in mortality in anterior wall MI patients, not treated with fibrinolytics, using zofenopril.[23] The largest study, the Fourth International Study of Infarct Survival (ISIS-4); randomized 58 050 AMI patients to receive either captopril or placebo within 24 h of presentation.[24] The reduction of mortality was seen in 5 weeks (7.2% versus 7.7%) in the captopril group. The majority of patients in this study were initially treated with fibrinolytic therapy. The GISSI-3 study also showed similar early benefit in mortality, which persisted in the higher-risk patients.[25] Unlike intravenous β-blockers, intravenous enalapril was associated with more hypotension and a trend towards higher mortality in patients enrolled in the prematurely terminated Cooperative New Scandinavian Enalapril Survival Study (CONSENSUS)-II trial.[26]

Angiotensin receptor blockers also inhibit the renin–angiotensin–aldosterone system. The Valsartan in Acute Myocardial Infarction (VALIANT) study compared captopril, valsartan and the combination in a large randomized trial of post-MI patients and left ventricular dysfunction.[27] The study showed that valsartan was as effective as captopril (HR 1.0, 95% CI 0.90–1.11, p = 0.98) but the addition of valsartan to captopril did not improve survival and increased adverse events. Valsartan had significantly reduced risks of angioedema. The Optimal Trial in Myocardial Infarction with Angiotensin II Antagonist Losartan (OPTIMAAL) trial randomized 5477 acute myocardial infarction patients with congestive heart failure to losartan or captopril therapy.[28] There was no statistical difference in mortality after 2.7 years (18% losartan, 16% captopril groups, RR 1.13, 95% CI 0.99–1.28, p = 0.07).

Table 7.2 Randomized trials of angiotensin converting enzyme inhibitors versus placebo in acute myocardial infarction

Study	Agent	Patients (n)	Duration	RR of death	p Value
ISIS-4	Captopril	58 050	35 days	0.93 (0.87–0.99)	0.02
GISSI-3	Lisinopril	19 394	42 days	0.88 (0.79–0.99)	0.03
CONSENSUS-II	Enalaprilat	6090	41–180 days	1.11 (0.93–1.29)	0.26
SAVE	Captopril	2231	42 months	0.81 (0.68–0.97)	0.02
AIRE	Ramipril	2006	15 months	0.73 (0.69–0.89)	0.002
TRACE	Trandolapril	1749	24–50 months	0.78 (0.70–0.86)	< 0.001

Recommendations

Therefore, it is clear that ACE inhibitors improve outcome when used early and continued long term in patients with AMI, especially those with left ventricular dysfunction. It is therefore recommended that ACE inhibitors be initiated early (within 24 h) in patients suffering AMI.[16] Short-acting agents such as captopril (6.25 mg initially with rapid titration to 50 mg TID) may be preferable for initial in-hospital titration. However, patients should be switched to adequate doses as tolerated of longer-acting agents for outpatient therapy to ensure compliance. The contraindications for ACE-inhibitor use are severe hypotension, known bilateral renal artery stenosis, acute renal failure and hypersensitivity to ACE inhibitors (angioedema). Caution should be exercised in patients with hypovolemia, hyperkalemia, hyponatremia and renal insufficiency. The major side-effects of renal insufficiency and hyperkalemia may need discontinuation or dose lowering. If patients develop intolerance to ACE inhibitors, they may be switched to selective angiotensin receptor blockers (ARBs).

CALCIUM CHANNEL BLOCKERS

The calcium channel in the cardiomyocytes and vascular smooth muscle cells regulates the influx of calcium across the cell membrane, affecting the plateau phase of the action potential. Calcium channel blockers in experimental models have shown various beneficial effects during ischemia, infarction and reperfusion. They have been shown to reduce ischemia by reducing myocardial oxygen demand, preserving metabolism of high-energy phosphates, reducing myocardial stunning and reperfusion injury, and possibly reducing platelet and neutrophil damage in the infarcted myocardium.

Despite the theoretical benefits of calcium channel blockers, they have not been shown to have conclusive clinical benefit in patients with AMI (Table 7.3).

Nifedipine is a dihydropyridine calcium channel blocker that has been extensively studied to treat cardiac conditions. Trials administering nifedipine early in patients with AMI have not been shown to improve outcome.[29,30] In patients treated with fibrinolytic therapy and nifedipine there was evidence of larger MI

Table 7.3 Randomized trials of calcium channel blockers in acute myocardial infarction

Study	Agent	Patients (n)	Duration	RR of death	p Value
TRENT	Nifedipine	4491	1 month	1.07 (0.86–1.34)	0.56
SPRINT II	Nifedipine	1358	6 months	1.33 (0.98–1.80)	0.09
DAVIT I	Verapamil	1436	6 months	0.91 (0.67–1.24)	ns
SPRINT I	Nifedipine	2276	10 months	1.07 (0.77–1.50)	0.42
DAVIT II	Verapamil	1775	16 months	0.80 (0.61–1.05)	0.11
MDPIT	Diltiazem	2466	25 months	1.02 (0.82–1.27)	ns

compared to controls.[31] Overall the use of nifedipine in patients with coronary artery disease has been questioned with the results of a meta-analysis showing increased mortality (HR 1.16, 95% CI 1.01–1.33).[32]

Diltiazem is a benzothiazepine calcium channel blocker that has been studied in randomized trials in patients with AMI. The Multicenter Diltiazem Post-Infarction Trial (MDPIT) randomized 2446 patients to diltiazem 240 mg/day or placebo for a mean of 25 months.[33] Although there was no reduction in mortality, cardiac events were reduced in patients with preserved left ventricular function. However, there was increased cardiac death and non-fatal MI in patients with impaired left ventricular function (ejection fraction < 40%). Gibson *et al.* reported a reduction in reinfarction and refractory angina after non-Q wave MI with the use of diltiazem.[34] The Incomplete Infarction Trial of European Research Collaborators Evaluation Prognosis post-Thrombolysis (INTERCEPT) trial studied patients who were treated with fibrinolysis for AMI and who did not have heart failure.[35] At 6-month follow-up, the occurrence of cardiac death, non-fatal MI or refractory ischemia was not reduced but a reduction was seen in the need for revascularization. Several smaller studies have also reported a reduction in reinfarction and recurrent ischemia with diltiazem in AMI patients treated with streptokinase or activase.[36,37]

Verapamil is a calcium channel blocker that has similar properties to those of diltiazem and has been studied in patients with AMI. The Danish Verapamil Infarction Trial I (DAVIT I) demonstrated a trend toward benefit of verapamil in non-reperfused AMI patients.[38] The DAVIT II study randomized patients to receive verapamil or placebo 7–15 days after an AMI. In patients without congestive heart failure there was significant reduction in reinfarction (9.4% vs. 12.7%) and mortality (7.7% vs. 11.8%).[39] The Calcium antagonist Reinfarction Italian Study (CRIS) in patients with AMI failed to show benefit of verapamil.[40] Smaller studies of AMI patients treated with fibrinolysis and verapamil did not show a difference in clinical outcome but there was an improvement in diastolic function and end-diastolic left ventricular volume.[41,42]

An early meta-analysis of the use of calcium channel blockers in AMI in the pre-fibrinolytic era reported a trend towards increased all-cause mortality (OR 1.06, 95% CI 0.96–1.18).[43]

Recommendations

With the available evidence, calcium channel blockers should not be used as first-line therapy in patients with AMI. In patients with non-ST segment elevation MI, a long-acting calcium channel blocker may be used to reduce ischemia and rein-farction.[16] However, it would be preferable to use β-blockers and ACE inhibitors first and add calcium channel blockers only if there is refractory ischemia, hypertension, rapid atrial fibrillation, or contraindications to β-blockers. Calcium channel blockers should not be used in patients with ST segment elevation MI, congestive heart failure and evidence of left ventricular systolic dysfunction.

NITRATES

Nitroglycerin is an organic nitrate that is converted to nitric oxide in the tissues. It then acts on the enzyme guanylate cyclase, which stimulates the synthesis of cGMP. It is a potent vasodilator that has been primarily used to treat angina since 1846.

Nitrates decrease the oxygen requirement of the heart by decreasing preload and afterload. They cause epicardial arterial dilatation with increased myocardial perfusion. They have also been shown to reduce infarct size in experimental models and increase collateral blood flow.[44] Because of the vasodilatory, anti-ischemic and endothelium-modulating properties, nitrates have been studied to treat AMI extensively.

A meta-analysis of smaller trials had reported that use of nitroglycerin or nitroprusside was associated with 35% reduction in mortality of AMI patients.[45] In the GISSI-3 trial of 18 895 AMI patients treated with aspirin (84%) and fibrinolysis (72%), there was no difference in outcome in the group of patients assigned to transdermal glyceryl trinitrate.[25] The definitive ISIS-4 trial of 58 050 AMI patients showed no significant benefits of oral mononitrate administration.[24] Both these trials, however, confirmed the safety of nitroglycerin use during AMI.

Recommendations

Routine use of nitrates in patients with AMI does not improve outcome. However, nitrates can be used initially in AMI patients for effective treatment of hypertension, refractory ischemia, or congestive heart failure. Intravenous nitroglycerin can be initiated in the acute setting and changed to oral therapy for chronic use if required.[16]

STATINS

HMG Coenzyme-A reductase inhibitors (statins) are potent agents that lower serum cholesterol levels effectively in patients. They have been shown to reduce death and cardiovascular events in the primary and secondary prevention setting in patients with hyperlipidemia.[46–51]

Statins have been demonstrated to have significant anti-inflammatory and other pleiotropic properties that are beneficial to patients at risk of cardiovascular events. They have been proposed to increase nitric oxide production, decrease endothelin-1, increase endogenous tissue plasminogen activator, decrease plasminogen activator inhibitor-1, decrease tissue factor, decrease platelet aggregation, reduce matrix met-alloproteinases, reduce inflammation, decrease C-reactive protein, increase collagen content and reduce lipid content in the atherosclerotic plaque.

Recently, statins have been studied in patients with AMI in the acute setting. The Myocardial Ischemia Reduction with Aggressive Cholesterol Lowering (MIRACL) trial randomized patients to receive high-dose atorvastatin or placebo after acute coronary syndrome and demonstrated significant reduction (17.4% vs. 14.8%,

$p = 0.048$) in composite cardiovascular events in 16 weeks.[52] The Pravastatin or Atorvastatin Evaluation and Infection Therapy – Thrombolysis in Myocardial Infarction-22 (PROVE-IT TIMI 22) study randomized 4162 patients to receive either 80 mg of atorvastatin or 40 mg of pravastatin in hospitalized patients' acute coronary syndrome.[53] At a mean 24-month follow-up, there was a significant 16% (95% CI 5–26%, $p = 0.005$) reduction in death and cardiovascular events (Figure 7.1). The mean low-density lipoprotein–cholesterol in the atorvastatin group was reduced to 62 mg/dl. The reduction in C-reactive protein levels was a more potent predictor of future events in this study than reduction in cholesterol.[54] Although statins have not been studied in patients with ST segment elevation MI undergoing reperfusion therapy, the results of studies in acute coronary syndromes can be extrapolated to these patients as well.

Recommendations

Statins should be initiated in all AMI patients if not contraindicated prior to hospital discharge, regardless of initial cholesterol measurement. There is preliminary evidence that the anti-inflammatory effects of statins occur much earlier than the lipid-lowering effects and, therefore, high-dose statins should be considered as early as possible after hospitalization.

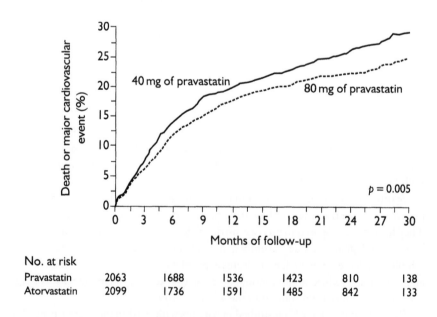

No. at risk						
Pravastatin	2063	1688	1536	1423	810	138
Atorvastatin	2099	1736	1591	1485	842	133

Figure 7.1 Kaplan–Meier estimates of the incidence of the primary endpoint of death or a cardiovascular event showing 16% reduction in events in the group treated with 80 mg of atorvastatin (from reference 53, with permission).

ADENOSINE

Adenosine is an endogenous purine nucleotide and a biproduct of adenosine monophosphate, which is found in all tissues of the body. It is primarily used as a vasodilator and an anti-arrhythmic to treat supraventricular tachycardia.

It has vasodilatory, antiadrenergic and negative chronotropic properties that potentially can reduce myocardial ischemia and infarction size. The vasodilatory effect is primarily at the level of resistance vessels, which may be important in improving tissue level circulation after epicardial reperfusion.

The Acute Myocardial Infarction Study of Adenosine (AMISTAD) trial randomized AMI patients treated with fibrinolysis to intravenous adenosine infusion or placebo. Patients treated with adenosine had smaller infarct size (reduced by 67%, $p = 0.014$) as measured by nuclear imaging at 6 days in the subgroup of patients with anterior MI.[55] There was no reduction in infarct size in non-anterior MI patients. The AMISTAD II trial randomized 236 patients with anterior MI treated with fibrinolysis to two doses of adenosine (AMISTAD II). There was no significant difference between adenosine versus placebo, but the higher-dose patients had reduction in infarct size with a trend towards event reduction.[56] Marzilli *et al.* reported significantly improved epicardial TIMI-3 flow and reduced adverse events in 54 patients undergoing AMI PCI with intracoronary bolus injection of adenosine compared to saline.[57] A study of 79 patients undergoing PCI for AMI receiving 20 min of intracoronary adenosine infusion reported reduced reperfusion injury and better QRS-derived infarct score compared to 200 historical controls.[58] Another study of an adenosine agonist in 311 patients undergoing primary percutaneous coronary intervention reported no reduction in final infarct size.[59] The ATTenuation by Adenosine of Cardiac Complication (ATTACC) study used 6 h of adenosine infusion as an adjunctive treatment with fibrinolysis in 608 patients.[60] There was no improvement in left ventricular function but there was a trend towards improved mortality at 12 months in the patients treated with adenosine.

Recommendations

There is insufficient evidence to recommend routine intravenous infusion of adenosine in patients treated with reperfusion therapy for AMI. There is reasonable evidence to use intracoronary boluses (100–4000 μg) of adenosine after primary percutaneous reperfusion of an infarct-related artery to improve microvascular flow.

GLUCOSE–INSULIN–POTASSIUM

Glucose and insulin increase glycolytic ATP synthesis during hypoxia. Metabolic protection of ischemic myocardium can be facilitated by ATP generation through the anaerobic glycolytic pathway and suppression of myocardial fatty acid uptake.[61] Insulin also facilitates glucose and potassium uptake into cells, potentially reducing ischemic damage and arrhythmia.[62] Insulin has been shown to have an anti-inflammatory and profibrinolytic effect in patients with AMI.[63]

Therefore, glucose–insulin–potassium (GIK) has been studied in many smaller trials of AMI. A meta-analysis of 1900 AMI patients treated with GIK in the pre-fibrinolytic era reported 28% reduction in in-hospital mortality.[64] The Estudios Cardiologicos Latino-America (ECLA) trial randomized 407 patients with AMI, 72% treated with reperfusion therapy, to GIK or placebo.[65] The trial demonstrated a trend towards a mortality benefit in the overall population in the GIK group and a statistically significant mortality benefit in the subgroup undergoing reperfusion therapy (RR 0.34, 95% CI 0.5–0.8, $p = 0.008$). The DIGAMI study randomized 306 diabetic patients with AMI and demonstrated reduction in 1-year mortality with glucose–insulin versus conventional therapy (18.6% vs. 26.1%, $p = 0.03$).[66] The Polish GIK trial found no benefit of low-dose GIK in AMI patients.[67] The Dutch Glucose–Insulin–Potassium Study (GIPS) also found no significant benefit of GIK in patients undergoing primary PCI but reported a benefit in the subgroup presenting with Killip class I.[68]

The definitive CREATE-ECLA was a multinational trial that randomized 20 201 patients to receive high-dose GIK (25% glucose, 50 U/l regular insulin and 80 mEq/l of potassium infused at 1.5 ml/kg per h) or placebo in patients admitted with ST elevation MI and treated with reperfusion (74% fibrinolysis, and 9% primary PCI).[69] There was no difference in mortality at 30 days between the groups (9.7% vs. 10.0%, HR 1.03, 95% CI 0.95–1.13, $p = 0.45$). There was no difference in the rates of cardiac arrest, cardiogenic shock, heart failure or reinfarction between the groups. There was more hyperkalemia, phlebitis and symptomatic hypoglycemia in the GIK group. On predefined subgroup analysis there was no improvement in outcome in any of the subgroups treated with GIK (Figure 7.2).

Recommendations

Although earlier trials and meta-analyses suggested benefit with GIK in AMI patients, the large definitive CREATE-ECLA trial demonstrated no benefit with this therapy. Therefore, GIK is not recommended to treat unselected AMI patients undergoing reperfusion therapy. Diabetic patients, however, need aggressive glucose control during MI to reduce morbidity and may benefit from continuous insulin infusion.

OTHER ADJUNCTIVE THERAPY

Sodium–hydrogen exchange inhibitors

These drugs decrease the influx of sodium into ischemic cells and this leads to less calcium that can be exchanged for the sodium going into the cell, potentially preserving cell metabolism and preventing necrosis. Experimental studies with cariporide reduced infarct size by 55% in coronary occlusion reperfusion rabbit models.[70] Rupprecht et al. demonstrated reduction in infarct size in patients

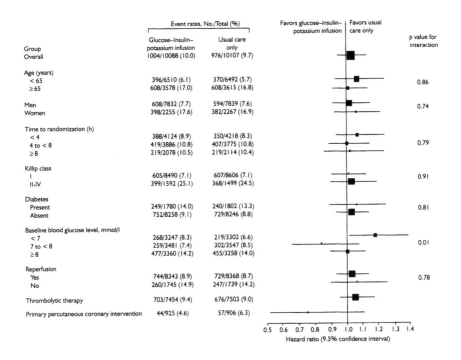

Group	Event rates, No./Total (%)				
	Glucose–Insulin–potassium infusion	Usual care only			p value for interaction
Overall	1004/10088 (10.0)	976/10107 (9.7)			
Age (years)					
< 65	396/6510 (6.1)	370/6492 (5.7)			0.86
≥ 65	608/3578 (17.0)	608/3615 (16.8)			
Men	608/7832 (7.7)	594/7839 (7.6)			0.74
Women	398/2255 (17.6)	382/2267 (16.9)			
Time to randomization (h)					
< 4	388/4124 (8.9)	350/4218 (8.3)			
4 to < 8	419/3886 (10.8)	407/3775 (10.8)			0.79
≥ 8	219/2078 (10.5)	219/2114 (10.4)			
Killip class					
I	605/8490 (7.1)	607/8606 (7.1)			0.91
II–IV	399/1592 (25.1)	368/1499 (24.5)			
Diabetes					
Present	249/1780 (14.0)	240/1802 (13.3)			0.81
Absent	752/8258 (9.1)	729/8246 (8.8)			
Baseline blood glucose level, mmol/l					
< 7	268/3247 (8.3)	219/3302 (6.6)			
7 to < 8	259/3481 (7.4)	302/3547 (8.5)			0.01
≥ 8	477/3360 (14.2)	455/3258 (14.0)			
Reperfusion					
Yes	744/8343 (8.9)	729/8368 (8.7)			0.78
No	260/1745 (14.9)	247/1739 (14.2)			
Thrombolytic therapy	703/7454 (9.4)	676/7503 (9.0)			
Primary percutaneous coronary intervention	44/925 (4.6)	57/906 (6.3)			

Favors glucose–insulin–potassium infusion | Favors usual care only

0.5 0.6 0.7 0.8 0.9 1.0 1.1 1.2 1.3 1.4
Hazard ratio (9.5% confidence interval)

Figure 7.2 Death at 30 days in the subgroups showing no significant benefit of glucose–insulin–potassium in any of the subgroups (from reference 69, with permission).

undergoing primary percutaneous coronary intervention using intravenous cariporide.[71] The Guard During Ischemia against Necrosis (GUARDIAN) trial investigated various doses of cariporide in patients with acute coronary syndrome or undergoing coronary artery bypass graft (CABG).[72] There was no difference in infarct size with cariporide in the overall study but patients undergoing CABG had reduced myocardial infarction. The ESCAMI trial randomized 1411 patients with AMI to eniporide versus placebo. There was no reduction in infarct size with eniporide in this study but there was a trend towards increased mortality and stroke.[73]

Therefore, until further studies show benefit, this class of drugs is not recommended to treat patients undergoing reperfusion for AMI.

Complement inhibitors

Complement, when activated during myocardial ischemia and reperfusion, contributes to injury to the myocardium. Complement inhibition therefore has potential to reduce reperfusion injury in patients with AMI. Pexelizumab is a specific C5 complement inhibitor that has been tested in randomized studies of AMI. When tested in patients undergoing coronary bypass surgery, it was shown to

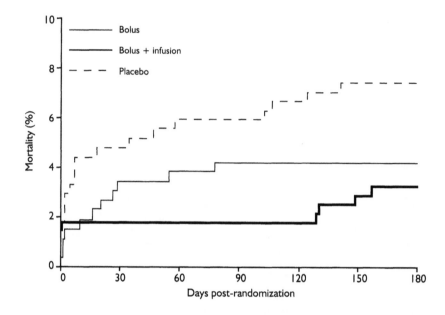

Figure 7.3 Kaplan–Meier survival curves at 6 months in the COMMA trial showing reduced mortality in patients receiving pexelizumab (from reference 76, with permission).

reduce the combined endpoint of death and MI (RR 0.82, 95% CI 0.68–0.99, $p = 0.03$).[74] The COMPLY trial randomly assigned 943 AMI patients receiving fibrinolysis with pexelizumab bolus, bolus plus infusion, or placebo. There was no difference in infarct size between the groups or the composite endpoint of death, congestive heart failure, shock, or stroke.[75] The COMMA study randomized 960 patients undergoing primary percutaneous coronary intervention similarly to pexelizumab bolus, bolus plus infusion, or placebo. There was no significant difference in the primary outcome of infarct size.[76] However, the patients receiving pexelizumab had significantly lower mortality (1.8% vs. 5.9%, $p = 0.014$) (Figure 7.3). There is no clear explanation for this result, but a phase III randomized study is underway to test this benefit further.

REFERENCES

1. Yusuf S, Reddy S, Ounpuu S, et al. Global burden of cardiovascular diseases, part I: general considerations, the epidemiological transition, risk factors, and impact of urbanization. Circulation 2001; 104: 2746–53

2. DeWood MA, Spores J, Notske R, et al. Prevalence of total coronary occlusion during the early hours of transmural myocardial infarction. N Engl J Med 1980; 303: 897–902

3. Fibrinolytic Therapy Trialists' (FTT) Collaborative Group. Indications for fibrinolytic therapy in suspected acute myocardial infarction: collaborative overview of early

mortality and major morbidity results from all randomised trials of more than 1000 patients. Lancet 1994; 343: 311–22

4. Weaver WD, Peberdy MA. Defibrillators in public places – one step closer to home. N Engl J Med 2002; 347: 1223–4

5. ISIS-1 (First International Study of Infarct Survival. Randomised trial of intravenous atenolol among 16 027 cases of suspected acute myocardial infarction: ISIS-1. First International Study of Infarct Survival Collaborative Group. Lancet 1986; 2: 57–66

6. The effects of tissue plasminogen activator, streptokinase, or both on coronary-artery patency, ventricular function, and survival after acute myocardial infarction. The GUSTO Angiographic Investigators. N Engl J Med 1993; 329: 1615–22

7. Yusuf S, Sleight P, Rossi P, et al. Reduction in infarct size, arrhythmia and chest pain by early intravenous beta blockade in suspected myocardial infarction. Circulation 1983; 67: 132–41

8. Hammerman H, Kloner RA, Briggs L, et al. Enhancement of salvage of reperfused myocardium by early beta blockade (timolol). J Am Coll Cardiol 1984; 3: 1438–43

9. The International Collaborative Study Group. Reduction of infarct size with the early use of timolol in acute myocardial infarction. N Engl J Med 1984; 310: 9–15

10. Hjalmarson A, Elmfield D, Herlitz J, et al. Effect on mortality of metoprolol in acute myocardial infarction: a double blind randomized trial. Lancet 1981; 2: 823–7

11. Beta-Blocker Heart Attack Trial Research Group. A randomized trial of propanolol in patients with acute myocardial infarction. Mortality results. J Am Med Assoc 1982; 247: 1707–14

12. The Norwegian Multicenter Study Group. Timolol-induced reduction in mortality and reinfarction in patients surviving acute myocardial infarction. N Engl J Med 1981; 304: 801–7

13. The MIAMI Trial Research Group. Metoprolol in acute myocardial infarction (MIAMI). A randomized placebo-controlled international trial. Eur Heart J 1985; 6: 199–226

14. Roberts R, Rogers WJ, Mueller HS, et al. Immediate versus deferred beta-blockade following thrombolytic therapy in patients with acute myocardial infarction. Results of the Thrombolysis in Myocardial Infarction (TIMI) II-B Study. Circulation 1991; 83: 422–37

15. Effect of carvedilol on outcome after myocardial infarction in patients with left ventricular dysfunction: the CAPRICORN randomized trial. Lancet 2001; 357: 1385–90

16. Antman EM, Anbe DT, Armstrong PW, et al. ACC/AHA guidelines for the management of patients with ST elevation myocardial infarction. A report of the American College of Cardiology/American Heart Association Task Force on Practice Guidelines (Writing Committee on Management to Revise the 1999 Guidelines for Management of Patients With Acute Myocardial Infarction). J Am Coll Cardiol 2004; 44: 671–719

17. The SOLVD Investigators. Effect of enalapril on survival in patients with reduced left ventricular ejection fractions and congestive heart failure. The SOLVD Investigators. N Engl J Med 1991; 325: 293–302

18. Cohn JN, Johnson G, Ziesche S, et al. A comparison of enalapril with hydralazine-isosorbide dinitrate in the treatment of chronic congestive heart failure. N Engl J Med 1991; 325: 303–10

19. Jeremy RW, Allman KC, Bautovitch G, Harris PJ. Patterns of left ventricular dilation during the six months after myocardial infarction. J Am Coll Cardiol 1989; 13: 304–10

20. Pfeffer MA, Braunwald E, Moye LA, et al. Effect of captopril on mortality and morbidity in patients with left ventricular dysfunction after myocardial infarction. Results of the

survival and ventricular enlargement trial. The SAVE Investigators. N Engl J Med 1992; 327: 669–77

21. The AIRE Study Investigators. Effect of ramipril on mortality and morbidity of survivors of acute myocardial infarction with clinical evidence of heart failure. The Acute Infarction Ramipril Efficacy (AIRE) study investigators. Lancet 1993; 342: 821–8

22. Kober L, Torp-Pederson C, Carlsen JE, et al. A clinical trial of the angiotensin-converting-enzyme inhibitor trandolapril in patients with left ventricular dysfunction after myocardial infarction. Trandolapril Cardiac Evaluation (TRACE) Study Group. N Engl J Med 1995; 333: 1670–6

23. Ambrosioni E, Borghi C, Magnani B. The effect of the angiotensin-converting-enzyme inhibitor zofenopril on mortality and morbidity after anterior myocardial infarction. The Survival of Myocardial Infarction Long-Term Evaluation (SMILE) Study Investigators. N Engl J Med 1995; 332: 80–5

24. ISIS-4 (Fourth International Study of Infarct Survival) Collaborative Group. ISIS-4: a randomised factorial trial assessing early oral captopril, oral mononitrate, and intravenous magnesium sulphate in 58 050 patients with suspected acute myocardial infarction. Lancet 1995; 345: 669–85

25. Gruppo Italiano per lo Studio della Sopravvivenza nell'infarto Miocardico. GISSI-3: effects of lisinopril and transdermal glyceryl trinitrate singly and together on 6-week mortality and ventricular function after acute myocardial infarction. Lancet 1994; 343: 1115–22

26. Swedberg K, Held P, Kjekshus J, Rasmussen K, Ryden L, Wedel H. Effects of the early administration of enalapril on mortality in patients with acute myocardial infarction. Results of the Cooperative New Scandinavian Enalapril Survival Study II (CONSEN-SUS II). N Engl J Med 1992; 327: 678–84

27. Pfeffer MA, McMurray JJ, Velasueez EJ, et al. Valsartan, captopril, or both in myocardial infarction complicated by heart failure, left ventricular dysfunction, or both. N Engl J Med 2003; 349: 1893–906

28. Dickstein K, Kjekshus J; OPTIMAAL Steering committee. Effect of losartan and captopril on mortality and morbidity in high-risk patients after acute myocardial infarction: the OPTIMAAL randomized trial. Optimal Trial in Myocardial Infarction with Angiotensin II Antagonist Losartan. Lancet 2002; 360: 752–60

29. Wilcox RG, Hampton JR, Banks DC, et al. Trial of early nifedipine in acute myocardial infarction: the Trent study. Br Med J 1986; 293: 1204–8

30. Secondary prevention reinfarction Israeli nifedipine trial (SPRINT). A randomized intervention trial of nifedipine in patients with acute myocardial infarction. The Israeli Sprint Study Group. Eur Heart J 1988; 9: 354–64

31. Erbel R, Pop T, Meinertz T, et al. Combination of calcium channel blocker and thrombolytic therapy in acute myocardial infarction. Am Heart J 1988; 115: 529–38

32. Furberg CD, Psaty BM, Meyer JV. Nifedipine. Dose-related increase in mortality in patients with coronary heart disease. Circulation 1995; 92: 1326–31

33. The Multicenter Diltiazem Postinfarction Trial Research Group (MDPIT). The effect of diltiazem on mortality and reinfarction after myocardial infarction. N Engl J Med 1988; 319: 385–92

34. Gibson RS, Boden WE, Theroux P, et al. Diltiazem and reinfarction in patients with non-Q-wave myocardial infarction. Results of a double-blind, randomized, multicenter trial. N Engl J Med 1986; 315: 423–9

35. Boden WE, van Gilst WH, Scheldewaert RG, et al. Diltiazem in acute myocardial infarction treated with thrombolytic agents: a randomised placebo-controlled trial.

Incomplete Infarction Trial of European Research Collaborators Evaluating Prognosis po ST Thrombolysis (INTERCEPT). Lancet 2000; 355: 1751–6

36. Nicolau JC, Ramires JA, Maggioni AP, et al. Diltiazem improves left ventricular systolic function following acute myocardial infarction treated with streptokinase. The Calcium Antagonist in Reperfusion Study (CARES) Group. Am J Cardiol 1996; 78: 1049–52

37. Theroux P, Gregoire J, Chin C, Pelletier G, de Guise P, Juneau M. Intravenous diltiazem in acute myocardial infarction. Diltiazem as adjunctive therapy to activase (DATA) trial. J Am Coll Cardiol 1998; 32: 620–8

38. The Danish Study Group on Verapamil in Myocardial Infarction. Verapamil in acute myocardial infarction: the Danish Verapamil Infarction Trial I (DAVIT I). Eur Heart J 1984; 5: 516–28

39. The Danish Study Group on Verapamil in Myocardial Infarction. Effects of verapamil on mortality and major events after acute myocardial infarction: the Danish Verapamil Infarction Trial II (DAVIT II). Am J Cardiol 1990; 66: 779–85

40. Rengo F, Carbonin P, Pahor M, et al. A controlled trial of verapamil in patients after acute myocardial infarction: results of the calcium antagonist reinfarction Italian study (CRIS). Am J Cardiol 1996; 77: 365–9

41. Natale E, Tubaro M, Di Marcotullio G, et al. The effect of verapamil on left ventricular remodelling and diastolic function after acute myocardial infarction (the Verapamil Infarction Study on Remodelling and Relaxation – VISOR). Cardiovasc Drugs Ther 1999; 13: 315–24

42. Marangelli V, Memmola C, Brigiani MS, et al. Early administration of verapamil after thrombolysis in acute anterior myocardial infarction. Effect on left ventricular remodeling and clinical outcome. VAMI Study Group. Verapamil Acute Myocardial Infarction. Italian Heart J 2000; 1: 336–43

43. Held PH, Yusuf S, Furberg CD. Calcium channel blockers in acute myocardial infarction and unstable angina: an overview. Br Med J 1989; 299: 1187–92

44. Jugdutt BI, Becker LC, Hutchins GM, Bulkley BH, Reid PR, Kallman CH. Effect of intravenous nitroglycerin on collateral blood flow and infarct size in the conscious dog. Circulation 1981; 63: 17–28

45. Yusuf S, Collins R, MacMahon S, Peto R. Effect of intravenous nitrates on mortality in acute myocardial infarction: an overview of the randomised trials. Lancet 1988; 1: 1088–92

46. 4S Investigators. Randomised trial of cholesterol lowering in 4444 patients with coronary heart disease: the Scandinavian Simvastatin Survival Study (4S). Lancet 1994; 344: 1383–9

47. Shepard J, Cobbe SM, Ford I, et al. Prevention of coronary heart disease with pravastatin in men with hypercholesterolemia. West of Scotland Coronary Prevention Study Group. N Engl J Med 1995; 333: 1301–7

48. Sacks FM, Pfeffer MA, Moye LA, et al. The effect of pravastatin on coronary events after myocardial infarction in patients with average cholesterol levels. Cholesterol and Recurrent Event Trial investigators. N Engl J Med 1996; 335: 1001–9

49. The long term Intervention with Pravastatin in Ischemic Disease (LIPID) Study Group. Prevention of cardiovascular events and death with pravastatin in patients with coronary heart disease and a broad range of initial cholesterol levels. N Engl J Med 1998; 339: 1349–57

50. Collins R, Armitage J, Parish S, Sleight P, Peto R; Heart Protection Study Collaborative Group. MRC/BHF Heart Protection Study of cholesterol-lowering with simvastatin in 20,536 high-risk individuals. A randomized placebo-controlled trial. Lancet 2002; 360: 7–22

51. Sever PS, Dahlof B, Poulter NR, et al.; ASCOT investigators. Prevention of coronary and stroke events with atorvastatin in hypertensive patients who have average or lower-than-average cholesterol concentrations, in the Anglo-Scandinavian Cardiac Outcomes Trial – Lipid Lowering Arm (ASCOT-LLA): a multicentre randomised controlled trial. Lancet 2003; 361: 1149–58

52. Schwartz GG, Olsson AG, Ezekowitz M, et al. Myocardial Ischemia Reduction with Aggressive Cholesterol Lowering (MIRACL) Study Investigators. Effects of atorvastatin on early recurrent ischemic events in acute coronary syndromes: the MIRACL study: a randomized controlled trial. J Am Med Assoc 2001; 285: 1711–18

53. Cannon CP, Braunwald E, McCabe CH, et al. Comparison of intensive and moderate lipid lowering with statins after acute coronary syndromes. Pravastatin or Atorvastatin Evaluation and Infection Therapy – Thrombolysis in Myocardial Infarction 22 Investigators. N Engl J Med 2004; 350: 1495–504

54. Ridker PM, Cannon CP, Morrow D, et al. Pravastatin or Atorvastatin Evaluation and Infection Therapy – Thrombolysis in Myocardial Infarction 22 Investigators. C-reactive protein levels and outcome after statin therapy. N Engl J Med 2005; 352: 20–8

55. Mahaffey KW, Puma JA, Barbagelata NA, et al. Adenosine as an adjunct to thrombolytic therapy for acute myocardial infarction: results of a multicenter, randomized, placebo-controlled trial: the Acute Myocardial Infarction STudy of ADenosine (AMISTAD) trial. J Am Coll Cardiol 1999; 34: 1711–20

56. Ross A, Gibbons R, Kloner RA, et al. Acute myocardial Infarction Study of Adenosine (AMISTAD II). J Am Coll Cardiol 2005; 45: 1775–80

57. Marzilli M, Orsini E, Marraccini P, Testa R. Beneficial effects of intracoronary adenosine as an adjunct to primary angioplasty in acute myocardial infarction. Circulation 2000; 101: 2154–9

58. Claeys MJ, Bosmans J, De Ceuninck M, et al. Effect of intracoronary adenosine infusion during coronary intervention on myocardial reperfusion injury in patients with acute myocardial infarction. Am J Cardiol 2004; 94: 9–13

59. Kopecky SL, Aviles RJ, Bell MR, et al. A randomized, double-blinded, placebo-controlled, dose-ranging study measuring the effect of an adenosine agonist on infarct size reduction in patients undergoing primary percutaneous transluminal coronary angioplasty: the ADMIRE study. Am Heart J 2003; 146: 146–52

60. Quintana M, Hjemdahl P, Sollevi A, et al. Left ventricular function and cardiovascular events following adjuvant therapy with adenosine in acute myocardial infarction treated with thrombolysis, results of the ATTenuation by Adenosine of Cardiac Complication (ATTACC) study. Eur J Clin Pharmacol 2003; 59: 1–9

61. Cave AC, Ingwall JS, Friedrich J, et al. ATP synthesis during low-flow ischemia: influence of increased glycolytic substrate. Circulation 2000; 101: 2090–6

62. Sybers HD, Maroko PR, Asraf M, Libby P, Braunwald E. The effect of glucose–insulin–potassium on cardiac ultrastructure following experimental coronary occlusion. Am J Pathol 1973; 70: 410–20

63. Chaudhuri A, Janicke D, Wilson MF, et al. Anti-inflammatory and profibrinolytic effect of insulin in acute ST segment-elevation myocardial infarction. Circulation 2004; 109: 849–54

64. Fath-Ordoubadi F, Beatt KJ. Glucose–insulin–potassium therapy for treatment of acute myocardial infarction: an overview of randomized placebo-controlled trials. Circulation 1997; 96: 1152–6

65. Diaz R, Paolasso EA, Piegas LS, et al. Metabolic modulation of acute myocardial infarction. The ECLA (Estudios Cardiologicos Latinoamerica) Collaborative Group. Circulation 1998; 98: 2227–34

66. Malmberg K, Ryden L, Efendic S, et al. Randomized trial of insulin–glucose infusion followed by subcutaneous insulin treatment in diabetic patients with acute myocardial infarction (DIGAMI study): effects on mortality at 1 year. J Am Coll Cardiol 1995; 26: 57–65

67. Ceremuzynski L, Budaj A, Czepiel A, et al. Low-dose glucose–insulin–potassium is ineffective in acute myocardial infarction: results of a randomized multicenter Pol-GIK trial. Cardiovasc Drugs Ther 1999; 13: 191–200

68. van der Horst IC, Zijlstra F, van't Hof AW, et al.; Zwolle Infarct Study Group. Glucose–insulin–potassium infusion in patients treated with primary angioplasty for acute myocardial infarction: the Glucose–Insulin–Potassium Study: a randomized trial. J Am Coll Cardiol 2003; 42: 784–91

69. The CREATE-ECLA Trial Group Investigators. Effect of glucose–insulin–potassium infusion on mortality in patients with acute ST-segment elevation myocardial infarction. The CREATE-ECLA randomized controlled trial. J Am Med Assoc 2005; 293: 437–46

70. Hale SL, Kloner RA. Effect of combined K(ATP) channel activation and Na+/H+ exchange inhibition on infarct size in rabbits. Am J Physiol Heart Circ Physiol 2000; 279: H2673–7

71. Rupprecht HJ, vom Dahl J, Terres W, et al. Cardioprotective effects of the Na/H exchange inhibitor cariporide in patients with acute anterior myocardial infarction undergoing direct PTCA. Circulation 2000; 101: 2902–8

72. Theroux P, Chaitman BR, Danchin N, et al. Inhibition of the sodium–hydrogen exchanger with cariporide to prevent myocardial infarction in high-risk ischemic situation: main results of the GUARDIAN trial. Guard during ischemia against necrosis (GUARDIAN) investigators. Circulation 2000; 102: 3032–8

73. Zeymer U, Suryapratana H, Monassier JP, et al. The Na/H exchange inhibitor eniporide as an adjunct to early reperfusion therapy for acute myocardial infarction: results of the evaluation of the safety and cardioprotective effects of eniporide in acute myocardial infarction (ESCAMI) trial. J Am Coll Cardiol 2001; 38: 1644–50

74. Verrier ED, Shernan SK, Taylor KM, et al. Terminal complement blockade with pexelizumab during coronary artery bypass surgery requiring cardiopulmonary bypass: a randomized trial. J Am Med Assoc 2004; 291: 2319–27

75. Mahaffey KW, Granger CB, Nicolau JC, et al. Effect of pexelizumab, an anti-C5 complement antibody, as adjunctive therapy to fibrinolysis in acute myocardial infarction: the COMPlement inhibition in myocardial infarction treated with thrombolysis (COMPLY) trial. Circulation 2003; 108: 1176–83

76. Granger CB, Mahaffey KW, Weaver WD, et al. Pexelizumab, an anti-C5 complement antibody, as adjunctive therapy to primary percutaeous coronary intervention in acute myocardial infarction: the COMplement inhibition in Myocardial infarction treated with Angioplasty (COMMA) trial. Circulation 2003; 108: 1184–90

8

Evaluation of reperfusion in the treatment of acute myocardial infarction

Peter Klootwijk

INTRODUCTION

Assessment of the perfusion status of the myocardium in patients with an acute ST-elevation syndrome is mandatory for optimal guiding of reperfusion therapy as well as short- and long-term risk assessment. The traditional approach for the assessment of patients having an acute coronary syndrome is based on three criteria: assessment of clinical symptoms, electrocardiographic findings on the admission electrocardiogram (ECG) and measurements of biochemical markers. In the same instance, these criteria may provide easily available non-invasive methods for monitoring of the reperfusion status of the infarct-related vessel and related myocardium. Thus, assessment of reperfusion may include clinical markers such as resolution of symptoms, electrocardiographic markers, e.g. the occurrence of specific arrhythmias and normalization of the ST segments, contrast echocardiography and monitoring of specific cardiac proteins in plasma.[1–4] In this overview markers of reperfusion will be discussed with emphasis on the usefulness of the different electrocardiographic techniques for detection of reperfusion and patency of the infarct-related artery in patients with ST-elevation acute coronary syndrome.

CORONARY ANGIOGRAPHY AS THE 'GOLD STANDARD' FOR THE ASSESSMENT OF REPERFUSION

Coronary angiography is still regarded as the gold standard for the assessment of reperfusion of the infarct-related coronary artery following reperfusion therapy in patients with ST elevation myocardial infarction. However, it should be appreciated that angiography supplies only very momentary information on the status of the infarct-related vessel. As such, the rapidly changing dynamics of coronary blood flow in an injured vessel through active thrombus formation, clot lysis, distal embolization, vasoconstriction and vasodilatation cannot be assessed properly by this technique. Angiographic (re)perfusion assessment is still based on the Thrombolysis In Myocardial Infarction (TIMI) flow grade determination in the epicardial infarct-related artery.[5] TIMI flow grade is typically measured directly following percutaneous coronary intervention or 60–90 min following the administration of thrombolytic therapy. Classification is graded 0 to 3, where TIMI 0–1 refers to a functionally occluded coronary artery with absent or minimal antegrade coronary flow beyond the occlusion and incomplete filling of the distal coronary bed, TIMI 2 flow refers to a still reduced antegrade epicardial coronary flow but with a complete filling of the distal bed and TIMI 3 flow refers to normal epicardial coronary flow. Already in the early days of reperfusion therapy, it was demonstrated that TIMI flow grade, if assessed directly following reperfusion therapy, closely correlated with short- and long-term outcome.[6] As a consequence it is not surprising that the accuracy of other direct or surrogate markers for assessment of reperfusion of the infarct-related artery have always been validated based on their correlation with this angiographic 'gold standard'.[7] However, this 'gold standard' may be questioned as it reflects only epicardial restoration of blood flow but not reperfusion of the micro-vascular bed at the nutritive cellular level. Despite epicardial vessel patency, a significant number of patients may have a profound reduction in antegrade coronary blood flow with a patent infarct-related artery, referred to as the 'no-reflow phenomenon' which probably reflects microvascular dysfunction.[8] Outcome is comparable with patients who have TIMI 0–1 flow or worse.[9] The presence of collateral blood flow to the infarct-related artery and its related infarcted area may influence microvascular perfusion in a positive manner, whereas, for example, TIMI 3 flow of the infarct-related artery with serious damage of the distal microvascular bed may cause the opposite. Markers of reperfusion should therefore be related and validated not only to TIMI flow (reflecting only epicardial blood flow), but also to reperfusion of the distal microvascular bed of the infarct-related artery.

Methods that have been developed to assess (re)perfusion of the microvascular bed include TIMI frame count and the myocardial blush grade (or TIMI myocardial perfusion grade).[9–11] TIMI frame count may further stratify patients with TIMI 3 flow into those with incomplete and complete reperfusion at the microvascular level, the latter being related to a better long-term outcome. Myocardial blush grade, defined as the degree of contrast density in the infarct-related myocardium, appears to be a predictor of long-term mortality independent of Killip class, TIMI flow grade, left ventricular ejection fraction, and other clinical parameters.[9]

THE ELECTROCARDIOGRAM FOR THE EVALUATION OF REPERFUSION

In 1918, using coronary ligation in dogs as a model, Fred H. Smith was the first to demonstrate that ST segment elevation in the ECG was a sign of coronary occlusion.[12] One year later, James Herrick published the first ECG obtained during the clinical picture of a myocardial infarction.[13] Since then, the ECG has evolved into one of the most important non-invasive diagnostic techniques of today – cardiology.[14] It is now generally believed that ST segment deviation (elevation/-depression) reflects reversible myocardial ischemia, caused by (1) the differences in resting and depolarization potentials between the ischemic and healthy myocardium; and (2) ischemia-induced shortening of the action potential duration.[15] These changes cause a voltage gradient between normal and ischemic zones, leading to current flow between these regions (current of injury), which subsequently gives rise to ST segment elevation or depression on the surface ECG. ST segment elevation reflects transmural ischemia. Isolated ST segment depression generally reflects nontransmural ischemia. In the presence of ST segment elevation, ST segment depression may also occur as the equivalent of ST elevation, being its reciprocal in concurrent leads.

Depending on definitions, approximately 50% of acute myocardial infarction patients present with ST changes suggestive of transmural ischemia (ST deviations ≥ 0.1–0.2 mV). In the absence of reperfusion of the infarct-related artery, the ST deviation will gradually lessen over the next 24–48 h, owing to necrosis of myocytes with subsequent burnout of the electrical gradient. In contrast, resolution of the ST segment deviation following reperfusion, as demonstrated by coronary angiography, will occur with an almost 5-fold faster time course than the changes associated with the natural evolution of acute myocardial infarction without reperfusion.[16] Thus, in patients with a transmural myocardial infarction receiving reperfusion therapy, the speed and the amount of ST segment elevation resolution are valuable markers for assessing the reperfusion grade of the infarct-related artery.

Serial 12-lead ECG and ST segment recovery following reperfusion therapy

Many studies have evaluated the usefulness of ST segment recovery from static serial 12-lead ECGs for assessment of coronary perfusion status, thereby using coronary angiography as the gold standard.[1] In most instances, two or three sequential ECGs were compared, e.g. the earliest (but not always the most ischemic) ECG with the ECG at 60 and/or 180 min following the initiation of reperfusion therapy. One of the first valid studies in this field was performed by Clemmensen et al.[17] This study comprised 53 patients with an acute myocardial infarction treated with thrombolytic therapy. Two serial ECGs were recorded, one on admittance, the other approximately 180 min after thrombolytic therapy. Directly following the second ECG, angiographic perfusion status was assessed, using the TIMI classification at first injection of contrast. Reduction of the sum of the ST segment elevation of $\geq 20\%$ within a predefined time interval of 180 min rendered sensitivity and specificity of 88 and 80%, respectively, for ECG versus angiographic patency assessment. Absence of rapid ST segment recovery suggested persistent coronary occlusion.

Although the results of other early studies reported conflicting results, it has been well proven now that the speed and extent of the ST segment recovery directly relate to the accuracy of prediction of reperfusion and vessel patency as well as to prognosis (Figure 8.1).[18–20]

When focusing on coronary flow, patients with TIMI grade 3 flow appear to have a significantly greater amount of ST segment recovery than patients with

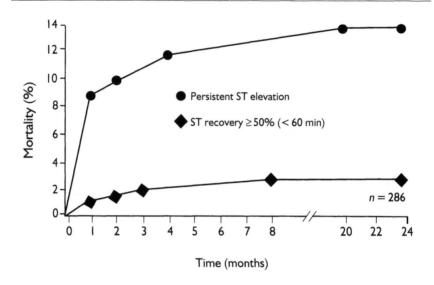

Figure 8.1   Presence or absence of ≥ 50% recovery of the sum of ST segment elevations 1 h after the initiation of thrombolytic treatment in 286 patients with an ST elevation myocardial infarction. ST elevations resolved rapidly within 1 h of treatment in 189 patients and persisted in 97 patients. Rapid resolution of ST elevations was associated with better long-term survival. Reproduced with permission from reference 18.

TIMI grade 2 flow (Figure 8.2).[21] Nevertheless, the probability of TIMI grade 3 flow is only 70–80% in patients with complete (≥70%) ST resolution (vs. approximately 90% for either TIMI grade 2 or 3 flow). Complete ST segment resolution may thus confirm that the infarct-related artery is patent, but it does not confirm that TIMI grade 3 flow is always present. On the other hand, if similar degrees of ST resolution are present, mortality appears to be similar in patients with TIMI grade 2 flow and TIMI grade 3 flow. This finding may be related to the quality of myocardial perfusion at the nutritive level. Related to this, van't Hof et al. evaluated myocardial blush grade correlating it with ST segment recovery.[9] It was demonstrated that, in patients who underwent primary angioplasty for acute myocardial infarction, myocardial blush grade could further risk stratify patients having TIMI 3 flow with an adverse outcome, who apparently did not have complete restoration of blood flow at the cellular level. Importantly, blush grade correlated better with the amount of ST segment resolution than with TIMI 3 flow. This suggests that ST segment recovery and blush grade both reflect myocardial flow at the nutritive level rather than at the epicardial flow level, thus predicting clinical outcome better than the assessment of epicardial vessel reperfusion and patency alone.

Many studies have demonstrated that complete ST segment recovery (≥70% within 1.5–3 h following the start of reperfusion therapy) is associated with a small infarct area and low short- and long-term mortality (1–2.5% at 30–35 days' follow-up, Figure 8.3).[20,22,23] Absence of ST segment recovery (<30% within 3h) may indicate failed reperfusion therapy, predicting a high mortality (e.g. 5.9–17.5% at

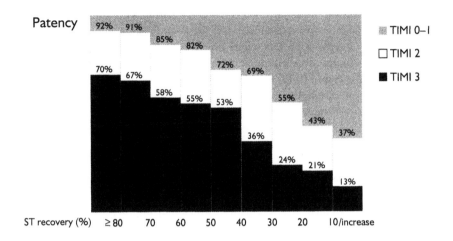

Figure 8.2 Comparison of baseline 12-lead ECG with 12-lead ECG 90 min following thrombolytic therapy. Incidence of TIMI 2 and 3 flow related to the sum ST segment resolution (sum of all ST segment elevations) in 447 patients, demonstrating a steady increase in patency rates with increase of ST segment resolution. Reproduced with permission from reference 21.

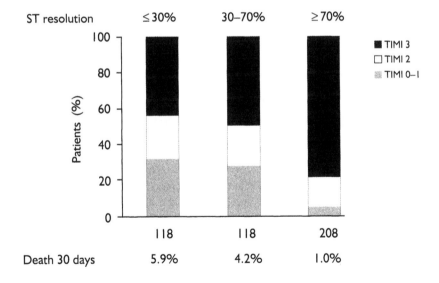

Figure 8.3 ST segment resolution in 444 patients with an ST elevation myocardial infarction receiving thrombolytic therapy. TIMI flow grade at 90 min after initiation of thrombolytic therapy versus per cent resolution of ST segment deviation and mortality at 30 days. Adapted from and reproduced with permission from reference 20.

30–35 days' follow-up). Recently, De Luca *et al.* reported on the additional value of incomplete resolution of concomitant ST segment depression in patients who demonstrated complete ST elevation resolution following primary angioplasty.[24] Incomplete resolution of concomitant ST segment depression appeared to be an independent predictor of 1-year mortality. Thus, in the setting of absence of ST segment recovery or incomplete resolution of concomitant ST segment depression despite complete ST elevation resolution, additional therapeutic interventions may be considered, despite a patent infarct-related epicardial coronary vessel, since these patients have more extensive myocardial damage.

Depending on the aims of reperfusion assessment, serial 12-lead ECG assessment may have major limitations. This method can only provide 'snapshot' information on the perfusion status of the myocardium. Close monitoring of the speed of the ST segment recovery pattern which may improve accurate prediction of the perfusion status of the infarct-related vessel is not possible.[25,26] Coronary reperfusion is a dynamic, rapidly changing process, which is often accompanied by intermittent or sustained reocclusion and cyclic flow changes. These dynamic changes may remain unrecognized if serial ECGs are used for monitoring. The time interval between the serial ECGs may be crucial for accurate detection of the true/actual peak of ST segment deviation. Underestimation of the degree of ST segment resolution and false assessment of the (sometimes short-lasting) first moment of reperfusion, with subsequent false interpretation of the coronary flow status, may be the result.

However, if the main goal is only risk assessment or evaluation of reperfusion regimens for study purposes, serial ECGs may suffice. In those instances where direct monitoring of the coronary perfusion and instant decision making is necessary, it may be more appropriate to use continuous ECG monitoring techniques, in order to avoid less accurate assessments of the perfusion status of the myocardium and erroneous decision making.

Continuous ECG monitoring for assessment of coronary perfusion in patients receiving reperfusion therapy

Through the years several continuous ECG monitoring techniques have been evaluated for the assessment of reperfusion and patency following reperfusion therapy. It has been demonstrated that these techniques have a stronger association with angiographic patency when compared to serial static ECGs.[27]

From a historical point of view, Holter ST segment recording was the first technique to monitor the ST segment continuously. As with serial ECG monitoring, this technique had major limitations. Only a restricted number of leads was available for monitoring, not always reflecting the area with maximal ST deviation. However, more importantly, even with the improvement of lead availability and digital recordings, Holter ST segment recording will always be limited by the fact that it can only provide information through retrospective data analysis (off-line analysis). This makes immediate feedback impossible and thus Holter techniques are not suitable for on-line monitoring of the perfusion status of the myocardium and immediate decision making. This may explain why only a few studies have been reported evaluating this technique for early reperfusion assessment. The two most representative studies, dating from before the era of computer-assisted ST monitoring systems, remain those from Hohnloser and Krucoff.[28,29] Both studies demonstrate that continuous ST segment recording may be used for retrospective ST segment recovery assessment.

Building on these experiences, in the early 1990s computer-assisted continuous multilead ECG monitoring techniques became available for real-time non-invasive reperfusion and patency assessment. Using continuous ECG sampling and averaging techniques, these techniques have proven to be of value for reperfusion assessment, offering a continuous real-time accurate measurement of the QRS complex and ST segment. Roughly speaking, two different approaches for computer-assisted ECG monitoring were developed: (1) continuous multilead ST segment monitoring, based on on-line monitoring of all 12 leads of the conventional 12-lead ECG, using either measurements of single leads or the summated ST segment level (nowadays many systems are available; the trendsetters were Mortara Instrument, Siemens Medical Electronics and Marquette);[30,31] and (2) continuous vectorcardiographic ECG monitoring, offering the possibility of studying the vectorcardiographic QRS complex and ST segment changes on-line and simultaneously the additional possibility of monitoring (vector-derived) 12 leads (Hewlett Packard/Agilent, Ortivus).[32] The majority of monitoring systems now offer the possibility of monitoring both the 12 leads individually as well as the continuous vectorcardiographic variables. The accuracy for predicting reperfusion and patency of the culprit coronary vessel is comparable for both digital monitoring methods.

As one of the first, Krucoff and co-workers reported on the presence of one episode of at least 50% ST segment recovery, the absence of recovery, or the recurrence of ST segment elevation, using continuous updated 12-lead computer-assisted ST monitoring. Reported sensitivity and specificity for prediction of occlusion were 64 and 90%, respectively, with predictive values for reperfusion and occlusion of 87 and 71%.[33]

Dellborg and colleagues were the first to report on vectorcardiographic assessment of reperfusion and patency using continuous vectorcardiographic monitoring. All of their studies used both QRS-vector difference and ST vector magnitude changes for prediction of the moment of reperfusion and vessel patency. By close eyeball observation of the ST segment behavior combined with observation of the QRS changes, sensitivity and specificity for prediction of patency at the moment of angiography were 94% and 80%, respectively, if a rapid change of both the QRS-vector difference and the ST vector magnitude was observed, ending in a steady state. If only the QRS-vector difference changes were used, sensitivity remained 94%, but specificity dropped to 40%.[34] Thus, compared to isolated ST segment monitoring, additional monitoring of the QRS vector seemed to increase the predictive performance of the device. However, in a later study of 96 patients using computer-assisted vectorcardiographic monitoring, more refined criteria were used and the angiographic assessment interval was fixed at 90 min as much as possible.

Sensitivity and specificity for identification of patency now were lower, 83% and 73%, respectively, and QRS-vector difference no longer contributed convincingly.[35]

ST segment patterns, peak ST segment deviation, speed and type of ST segment recovery

Taking into account both the speed and the amount of ST segment recovery, several distinct patterns of ST segment behavior following reperfusion therapy have been decribed:[30,32]

1. Rapid ST segment recovery without re-elevation
2. Rapid ST segment recovery following a delayed ST elevation peak
3. Persistent ST segment elevation without a recovery pattern
4. Rapid ST segment recovery followed by recurrent and persistent ST elevation
5. A delayed ST segment elevation peak followed by a rapid ST recovery and recurrent ST elevation

The first three patterns are direct markers for the status of the infarct-related artery: rapid ST recovery without re-elevation or a rapid ST recovery following a delayed ST elevation peak; both are highly suggestive of reperfusion of the infarct-related artery and myocardium.[26] In contrast, persistent ST segment elevation without a recovery pattern suggests persistent occlusion, provided that a significant level of ST elevation is present at the start of the monitoring period. However, rapid ST segment recovery followed by recurrent ST elevation or a delayed ST elevation peak followed by a rapid ST recovery and recurrent ST elevation may suggest unstable reperfusion. In the latter two instances patency assessment and correlation with 'snapshot' angiographic findings may be difficult.

The GUSTO-I ECG-ischemia monitoring sub-study evaluated the use of continuous vector-derived 12-lead, true 12-lead and 3-lead Holter ECG recording systems for prediction of reperfusion and patency in patients receiving thrombolytic therapy for an ST elevation myocardial infarction.[25] It demonstrated that non-invasive reperfusion and patency prediction using either of these continuous ECG recording techniques is feasible and can easily be used in clinical practice, particularly in patients with extensive initial ST segment elevation. If the combination of peak ST segment levels, speed of ST segment recovery and the type of ST recovery (with or without transient ST re-elevation) were taken into account, prediction of vessel status at the moment of angiography appeared to be 79–100% accurate in those patients with initially high ST levels. The latter is the group of patients having the greatest risk of adverse cardiac events and benefiting the most from reperfusion therapy and close observation of vessel status.[36] Although the three recording systems differed considerably in signal processing, no significant difference in accuracy of reperfusion and patency prediction was demonstrated among the three systems. The study demonstrated that tailoring of therapeutic strategies guided by computer-assisted continuous ECG monitoring techniques is feasible in patients with ST elevation myocardial infarction. This is illustrated by the following patient history (Figure 8.4):

A 50-year-old patient developed an acute inferior wall myocardial infarction 2 days before his scheduled elective coronary bypass surgery. During ambulance transfer to the hospital, thrombolytic therapy was initiated. On admission, the continuous ST monitoring device demonstrated persistent ST segment elevations in leads II, III, aVF, with concomitant ST segment depressions in leads I, aVL, V1-V5, suggesting persistent coronary occlusion (purple 12-lead ECG, moment A of the ST trend). Fifteen minutes later (moment B), the first moment of ST segment recovery occurred, directly followed by a recurrent temporary ST segment elevation (moment C). At this point the clinician decided to perform a percutaneous rescue intervention. However, just before transfer to the catherization laboratory, the ST segment level normalized and stabilized (green 12-lead ECG, and ST trend moment D). Therefore, the rescue intervention was

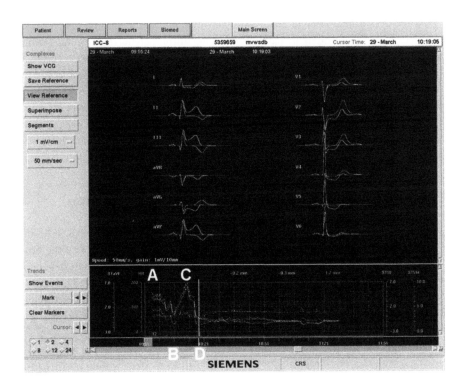

Figure 8.4 Continuous 12-lead ECG recording of a patient who developed an acute inferi-or wall myocardial infarction. For explanation see text. Colour code of 12-lead ECGs: purple ECG, reference ECG with ST elevations at admission; green ECG, ECG after stable reperfusion has occurred.

Trend curves at the bottom of the figure: green, heart rate; yellow, ST trend of lead III; blue, ST trend of lead aVF; orange, ST vector magnitude trend.

canceled and the patient underwent his bypass surgery 2 days later without any complication.

The changes of the ST segment are typical of a first moment of reperfusion of the culprit coronary artery at point B, followed by a short episode of 'reocclusion' at point C, most probably due to a washout and subsequent embolization of thrombus into the distal branches of the culprit coronary artery. Such 'reperfusion ST elevation peaks' may be mistakenly interpreted as harbingers of new coronary events still to come, but as in this patient these peaks are most commonly followed by permanent reperfusion of the infarcted area (moment D).

ST elevation reperfusion peaks and late recurrent ischemia following ST segment recovery

Early 'ST elevation reperfusion peaks', directly following ST segment recovery, occur in about 45–60% of patients and are associated with more extensive myocardial damage with subsequent higher mortality.[37–39] Compared to patients undergoing a primary percutaneous coronary intervention, these reperfusion peaks tend to occur more often in patients receiving thrombolytic therapy, suggesting more gradual washout and subsequent embolization of thombus in these patients.[40] Late recurrent ST segment shifts (either ST elevation or ST depression) 6–24 h following the start of reperfusion therapy can be observed in approximately 30% of patients with initial ST segment recovery suggestive of successful reperfusion. Similarly, as observed in patients with early 'ST elevation reperfusion peaks', these patients have higher mortality rates both at 30 days and at 1-year follow-up compared to those patients without recurrent ST shift.[41] The duration of the ST segment shift directly relates to subsequent mortality.

Time intervals and continuous ST segment monitoring

Assessment of reperfusion and patency of the infarct-related artery is relevant mainly during the first hours following reperfusion therapy. The longer is the time from onset of chest pain to the start of monitoring, the less ST segment deviation will be present at the start of monitoring, obscuring the true peak ST level at maximal acute ischemia. The amount of ST elevation present during monitoring is a major determinant of the accuracy of patency prediction: less ST deviation at the start of monitoring and during subsequent monitoring may result in less accurate prediction of vessel status.[25] The same is true for the delay from start of reperfusion therapy to the start of monitoring. In the GUSTO-I ECG-ischemia monitoring substudy the time from initiation of thrombolytic therapy to the first evidence of 50% ST segment recovery was less than 90 min in 75% of patients.[25] Therefore, in order to detect ST segment recovery, monitoring should be started early, preferably before the start of reperfusion therapy. If the start of monitoring is delayed and thrombolytic therapy has already been effective, the first moment of 50% ST recovery may not be properly recorded, which would result in false assessment of vessel status.

In a practical sense these observations indicate that ST segment monitoring should be initiated as soon as possible following arrival at the emergency ward. This will provide the operator with the optimal time window during which (sometimes very short-lasting) high ST segment levels can be detected, thus offering the optimal facilities to assess the true first moment of ST segment recovery and to predict vessel perfusion status most accurately.

Technical aspects of computer-assisted continuous ST segment monitoring

Computer-assisted continuous multilead and vectorcardiographic ECG-/ST segment monitoring use continuous ECG sampling and averaging techniques, which offer an accurate continuous real-time measurement of the QRS complex and ST segments. This remarkably improves the quality of the analysis compared to conventional ECG monitoring techniques. However, the user should appreciate the differences that exist between conventional ECG recording techniques and the various computer-assisted systems. Conventional techniques (e.g. Holter) measure the ST segment level from individual beats of the real-time ECG and subsequently average these measurements over fixed time intervals (generally 15 s to 1 min). In contrast, computer-assisted techniques average a number of ECG complexes in a preset time interval and subsequently calculate the ST segment level. Proper beat selection with exclusion of noisy beats can be done before averaging, resulting in more robust and accurate measurements. Conventional techniques will be more sensitive to abrupt ST segment changes, thus more easily triggering on minor ECG variations. In a noisy ECG environment, such a technique will also be most sensitive to noise. This is illustrated by the results of the GUSTO-I ECG-ischemia monitoring sub-study,[25] in which Holter ECG recording detected the moment of 50% ST segment recovery earlier (but not more accurately) than vectorcardiographic or 12-lead ECG-ischemia monitoring. It also detected more recurrent ST segment episodes (in 55% vs. 33% of patients). Thus, for correct interpretation of the signal, users should be aware of the characteristics of the device used. Adaptation of the ST analysis criteria to the individual characteristics of each device, to the demands of the user and to the aims for which monitoring is intended may result in optimal predictive performance and usefulness.

In general, computer-assisted ECG-/ST segment monitoring systems will render good-quality ECG recordings and analyses at a preset time interval of 1 min averaging. However, in some situations such as ECG-ischemia monitoring during coronary angiography or percutaneous coronary intervention, this time interval will be too long for detection of procedure-related short episodes of reperfusion or re-ischemia. A 15-second averaging may then be preferred. Opposite to this, the user should be aware of the fact that in case the sampling time interval of a computer-assisted system is set at an interval that is too long (e.g. 5 min instead of 1 min), the system will 'overlook' a short moment of reperfusion or re-ischemia, resulting in less accurate assessment of coronary vessel perfusion status.

Finally, ST segment monitoring of the single lead with the greatest initial ST segment shift will suffice in most patients with ST elevation myocardial infarction for detection of the first moment of reperfusion.[42] However, it should be appreciated that single-lead monitoring may not be appropriate for detection of recurrent ischemia in ST elevation myocardial infarction or non-ST elevation myocardial infarction, or in unstable angina patients. In these instances the site of the ischemic area may vary, depending on the flow balance of the coronary system, the degree of vessel injury and the duration and severity of ischemia.[41,43]

CARDIAC ARRHYTHMIAS AS MARKERS OF REPERFUSION

Cardiac arrhythmias may accompany coronary artery occlusion and reperfusion. Goldberg and colleagues were the first to report on the importance of early-occurring accelerated idioventricular rhythm (AIVR).[44] Wehrens et al. reported on the occurrence of ventricular arrhythmias during the first 10 min following reperfusion in 80–90% of patients, with an increase in ventricular premature complexes occurring in 48%, AIVR in 39% and bradycardia in 16% of patients.[40] This provides evidence that these arrhythmias are the direct consequence of restoration of coronary blood flow after a short-term occlusion.

AIVR is reported as the most reliable reperfusion arrhythmia.[40] Sensitivity and specificity fluctuate widely across studies depending on the reported incidence of AIVR, which may vary between 5 and 70%. Accuracy mainly depends on the timeframe and duration of arrhythmia monitoring. If AIVR occurs very early following reperfusion therapy, specificity and positive predictive values will be high, with values reported between 80 and 100%. However, if AIVR occurs late, correlation with reperfusion is lower, and as a consequence, sensitivity and negative predictive values are low as well. AIVR cannot be related to recurrent occlusion. Therefore, AIVR is not useful as a single marker of reperfusion, failed reperfusion or reocclusion.

Finally, the increased number of ventricular premature complexes, which may occur around the time of reperfusion, seems to be of limited predictive value, with a specificity of only 71%.[45] Non-sustained ventricular tachycardia and ventricular fibrillation have also been described, but are of less importance because of their infrequent appearance.[29,46]

ST SEGMENT MONITORING, CONTRAST ECHOCARDIOGRAPHY AND BIOCHEMICAL MARKERS FOR ASSESSING PERSISTENT OCCLUSION AND THE 'NO-REFLOW' PHENOMENON

ST segment recovery is closely related to the restoration of blood flow at the nutritive level, and thus a valuable marker of reperfusion. In fact the observation of such changes of the ST segment level indicate sufficient ST level amplitude and 'signal to noise ratio' for detecting a significant amount of ST segment changes with subsequent useful predictive values. Persistence of ST segment elevation is a different matter. In most instances this will indicate either persistent occlusion or, in the presence of a restored epicardial blood flow, the 'no-reflow phenomenon' which in fact reflects the absence of reperfusion at the nutritive myocardial level and is related to a poor prognosis.[22,47] However, persistence of ST segment elevation should not be confused with undocumented ('pseudo') absence of ST segment recovery. Undocumented ('pseudo') absence of ST segment recovery may not always reflect the absence of reperfusion. Confounding factors obscuring 'true' ST segment recovery may be insufficient ST elevation to detect ST recovery (low ST level amplitude and low 'signal to noise ratio') or unnoticed ST segment recovery, which already occurred before the start of ST segment monitoring. Taking this into account, it should be appreciated that ST segment monitoring may be less reliable for predicting persistent occlusion (GUSTO-I), although reocclusion following reperfusion can be predicted more accurately.[25]

In the instance of a suspected 'no-reflow phenomenon' ST segment monitoring might well be combined with myocardial contrast echocardiography and bio-chemical markers.[2,4] Already in the early 1990s, Ito et al. demonstrated that many patients with successful epicardial reperfusion had 'no reflow' at the level of the coronary microcirculation.[48] Myocardial contrast echocardiography appears to be especially useful for the assessment of the area at risk during acute coronary occlusion and for the detection of microvascular damage following reperfusion therapy causing the no reflow. If ST segment monitoring is inconclusive, the use of myocardial contrast echocardiography may result in an improvement of accurate assessment of the myocardial perfusion status at the microvascular/nutritive level. The technique is also useful for reliably differentiating between myocardial stunning and the 'no-reflow phenomenon'.

Several studies have investigated biochemical markers such as myoglobin and creatine kinase MB-fraction for prediction of reperfusion.[3,4] Recently, the ACC/AHA task force concluded that these markers can be useful for supportive evidence of reperfusion (class IIa recommendation).[49] The level of serum myoglobin is a sensitive marker of myocardial damage. When combined with clinical variables, myoglobin and/or creatine kinase MB may predict TIMI 2–3 flow accurately with reported probabilities of 85–90%.[3,4] In those instances where 'no reflow' of the infarct-related artery bed is suspected, peak myoglobin levels may contribute to accurate assessment of myocardial perfusion status if combined with ST segment monitoring and myocardial contrast echocardiography. However, these biochemical markers still have major limitations. In order to achieve accurate evaluation of the moment of reperfusion or absence of reperfusion, serial assays are necessary, but direct and on-line availability of these markers remains difficult.

COMBINED USE OF NON-INVASIVE MARKERS FOR ASSESSMENT OF MYOCARDIAL PERFUSION

The usefulness of ST segment monitoring, myocardial contrast echocardiography and biochemical markers for assessment of perfusion status may be underscored if they are used as isolated techniques only. The combined use of non-invasive markers for assessing reperfusion, reocclusion, persistent occlusion or 'no reflow' of the infarct-related artery has been evaluated extensively. Maas *et al.* combined baseline clinical descriptors with ST segment monitoring and demonstrated that the combination of high-risk clinical descriptors and high-risk ST variables more reliably identified a group in whom more aggressive and expensive therapies are warranted.[50] De Lemos *et al.* demonstrated that ST segment resolution, chest pain resolution and early washout of serum myoglobin could be used in an effective combination to improve early non-invasive identification of candidates for rescue percutaneous coronary intervention following thrombolytic therapy (Figure 8.5).[51]

Therefore, for daily practice purposes the clinician should combine baseline and clinical variables with easily available non-invasive tools as much as possible for optimal evaluation of reperfusion in the treatment of acute myocardial infarction.

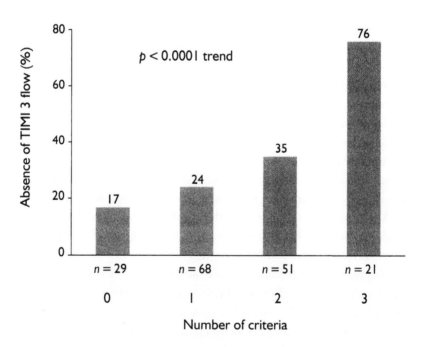

Figure 8.5 Correlation between absence of TIMI 3 flow and three non-invasive predictors of failed epicardial reperfusion following thrombolytic therapy, predictors being < 50% ST resolution at 90 min, 60 min/baseline ratio of myoglobin < 4 and persistent chest pain at the time of angiography. Adapted from and reproduced with permission from reference 51.

REFERENCES

1. Klootwijk P, Cobbaert C, Fioretti P, Kint PP, Simoons ML. Noninvasive assessment of reperfusion and reocclusion after thrombolysis in acute myocardial infarction. Am J Cardiol 1993; 72: 75G–84G

2. Sakuma T, Hayashi Y, Sumii K, Imazu M, Yamakido M. Prediction of short- and intermediate-term prognoses of patients with acute myocardial infarction using myocardial contrast echocardiography one day after recanalization. J Am Coll Cardiol 1998; 32: 890–7

3. Tanasijevic MJ, Cannon CP, Antman EM, et al. Myoglobin, creatine-kinase-MB and cardiac troponin-I 60-minute ratios predict infarct-related artery patency after thrombolysis for acute myocardial infarction: results from the Thrombolysis in Myocardial Infarction study (TIMI) 10B. J Am Coll Cardiol 1999; 34: 739–47

4. Iqbal MP, Kazmi KA, Mehboobali N, Rahbar A. Myoglobin – a marker of reperfusion and a prognostic indicator in patients with acute myocardial infarction. Clin Cardiol 2004; 27: 144–50

5. TIMI Study Group. The Thrombolysis in Myocardial Infarction (TIMI) trial. Phase I findings. N Engl J Med 1985; 312: 932–6

6. Ross AM, Coyne KS, Moreyra E, et al. Extended mortality benefit of early postinfarction reperfusion. GUSTO-I Angiographic Investigators. Global Utilization of Streptokinase and Tissue Plasminogen Activator for Occluded Coronary Arteries Trial. Circulation 1998; 97: 1549–56

7. Shah A, Wagner GS, Granger CB, et al. Prognostic implications of TIMI flow grade in the infarct related artery compared with continuous 12-lead ST segment resolution analysis. Reexamining the 'gold standard' for myocardial reperfusion assessment. J Am Coll Cardiol 2000; 35: 666–72

8. Rezkalla SH, Kloner RA. No-reflow phenomenon. Circulation 2002; 105: 656–62

9. van't Hof AW, Liem A, Suryapranata H, Hoorntje JC, de Boer MJ, Zijlstra F. Angiographic assessment of myocardial reperfusion in patients treated with primary angioplasty for acute myocardial infarction: myocardial blush grade. Zwolle Myocardial Infarction Study Group. Circulation 1998; 97: 2302–6

10. Gibson CM, Cannon CP, Murphy SA, Marble SJ, Barron HV, Braunwald E. Relationship of the TIMI myocardial perfusion grades, flow grades, frame count, and percutaneous coronary intervention to long-term outcomes after thrombolytic administration in acute myocardial infarction. Circulation 2002; 105: 1909–13

11. Dibra A, Mehilli J, Dirschinger J, et al. Thrombolysis in myocardial infarction myocardial perfusion grade in angiography correlates with myocardial salvage in patients with acute myocardial infarction treated with stenting or thrombolysis. J Am Coll Cardiol 2003; 41: 925–9

12. Smith FH. The ligation of coronary arteries with electrocardiographic study. Arch Intern Med 1918; 22: 8–15

13. Herrick JB. Thrombosis of the coronary arteries. J Am Med Assoc 1919; 72: 387

14. Fye WB. A history of the origin, evolution, and impact of electrocardiography. Am J Cardiol 1994; 73: 937–49

15. Vincent GM, Abildskov JA, Burgess MJ. Mechanisms of ischemic ST segment displacement. Evaluation by direct current recordings. Circulation 1977; 56: 559–66

16. Essen R, Merx W, Effert S. Spontaneous course of ST segment elevation in acute anterior myocardial infarction. Circulation 1979; 59: 105–12

17. Clemmensen P, Ohman EM, Sevilla DC, et al. Changes in standard electrocardiographic ST segment elevation predictive of successful reperfusion in acute myocardial infarction. Am J Cardiol 1990; 66: 1407–11

18. Barbash GI, Roth A, Hod H, et al. Rapid resolution of ST elevation and prediction of clinical outcome in patients undergoing thrombolysis with alteplase (recombinant tissue-type plasminogen activator): results of the Israeli Study of Early Intervention in Myocardial Infarction. Br Heart J 1990; 64: 241–7

19. Schroeder R, Dissmann R, Bruggemann T, et al. Extent of early ST segment elevation resolution: a simple but strong predictor of outcome in patients with acute myocardial infarction. J Am Coll Cardiol 1994; 24: 384–91

20. de Lemos JA, Antman EM, Giugliano RP, et al. ST segment resolution and infarct-related artery patency and flow after thrombolytic therapy. Thrombolysis in Myocardial Infarction (TIMI) 14 investigators. Am J Cardiol 2000; 85: 299–304

21. Zeymer U, Schroder R, Tebbe U, Molhoek GP, Wegscheider K, Neuhaus KL. Non-invasive detection of early infarct vessel patency by resolution of ST segment elevation in patients with thrombolysis for acute myocardial infarction; results of the angiographic substudy of the Hirudin for Improvement of Thrombolysis (HIT)-4 trial. Eur Heart J 2001; 22: 769–75

22. van't Hof AW, Liem A, de Boer MJ, Zijlstra F. Clinical value of 12-lead electro-cardiogram after successful reperfusion therapy for acute myocardial infarction. Zwolle Myocardial Infarction Study Group. Lancet 1997; 350: 615–19

23. Schroder K, Wegscheider K, Zeymer U, Tebbe U, Schroder R. Extent of ST segment deviation in a single electrocardiogram lead 90 min after thrombolysis as a predictor of medium-term mortality in acute myocardial infarction. Lancet 2001; 358: 1479–86

24. De Luca G, Maas AC, van't Hof AW, et al. Impact of ST segment depression resolution on mortality after successful mechanical reperfusion in patients with ST segment elevation acute myocardial infarction. Am J Cardiol 2005; 95: 234–6

25. Klootwijk P, Langer A, Meij S, et al. Non-invasive prediction of reperfusion and coronary artery patency by continuous ST segment monitoring in the GUSTO-I trial [published erratum appears in Eur Heart J 1996; 17: 1451] [see comments]. Eur Heart J 1996; 17: 689–98

26. Gibson CM, Karha J, Giugliano RP, et al. Association of the timing of ST segment resolution with TIMI myocardial perfusion grade in acute myocardial infarction. Am Heart J 2004; 147: 847–52

27. Veldkamp RF, Green CL, Wilkins ML, et al. Comparison of continuous ST segment recovery analysis with methods using static electrocardiograms for noninvasive patency assessment during acute myocardial infarction. Thrombolysis and Angioplasty in Myocardial Infarction (TAMI) 7 Study Group. Am J Cardiol 1994; 73: 1069–74

28. Krucoff MW, Green CE, Satler LF, et al. Noninvasive detection of coronary artery patency using continuous ST segment monitoring. Am J Cardiol 1986; 57: 916–22

29. Hohnloser SH, Zabel M, Kasper W, Meinertz T, Just H. Assessment of coronary artery patency after thrombolytic therapy: accurate prediction utilizing the combined analysis of three noninvasive markers. J Am Coll Cardiol 1991; 18: 44–9

30. Krucoff MW, Wagner NB, Pope JE, et al. The portable programmable microprocessor-driven real-time 12-lead electrocardiographic monitor: a preliminary report of a new device for the noninvasive detection of successful reperfusion or silent coronary reocclusion. Am J Cardiol 1990; 65: 143–8

31. Col J, Pirenne B, Decoster O, et al. Basic components and patterns of acute ischemia recovery assessed from continuous ST monitoring in acute myocardial infarction treated by thrombolytic therapy. J Electrocardiol 1994; 27 (Suppl): 241–8

32. Dellborg M, Riha M, Swedberg K. Dynamic QRS-complex and ST segment monitoring in acute myocardial infarction during recombinant tissue-type plasminogen activator therapy. The TEAHAT Study Group. Am J Cardiol 1991; 67: 343–9

33. Krucoff MW, Croll MA, Pope JE, et al. Continuous 12-lead ST segment recovery analysis in the TAMI 7 study. Performance of a noninvasive method for real-time detection of failed myocardial reperfusion. Circulation 1993; 88: 437–46

34. Dellborg M, Topol EJ, Swedberg K. Dynamic QRS complex and ST segment vectorcardiographic monitoring can identify vessel patency in patients with acute myocardial infarction treated with reperfusion therapy. Am Heart J 1991; 122: 943–8

35. Dellborg M, Steg PG, Simoons M, et al. Vectorcardiographic monitoring to assess early vessel patency after reperfusion therapy for acute myocardial infarction. Eur Heart J 1995; 16: 21–9

36. Willems JL, Willems RJ, Willems GM, Arnold AE, Van de WF, Verstraete M. Significance of initial ST segment elevation and depression for the management of thrombolytic therapy in acute myocardial infarction. European Cooperative Study Group for Recombinant Tissue-Type Plasminogen Activator. Circulation 1990; 82: 1147–58

37. Figueras J, Cortadellas J. Further elevation of the ST segment during the first hour of thrombolysis. A possible early marker of reperfusion. Eur Heart J 1995; 16: 1807–13

38. Yokoshiki H, Kohya T, Tateda K, Shishido T, Hirasawa K, Kitabatake A. Abrupt augmentation of ST segment elevation associated with successful reperfusion: a sign of diminished myocardial salvage. Am Heart J 1995; 130: 698–704

39. Johanson P, Wallentin L, Nilsson T, Bergstrand L, Lindahl B, Dellborg M. ST segment analyses and residual thrombi in the infarct-related artery: a report from the ASSENT PLUS ST monitoring substudy. Am Heart J 2004; 147: 853–8

40. Wehrens XH, Doevendans PA, Ophuis TJ, Wellens HJ. A comparison of electro-cardiographic changes during reperfusion of acute myocardial infarction by thrombolysis or percutaneous transluminal coronary angioplasty. Am Heart J 2000; 139: 430–6

41. Langer A, Krucoff MW, Klootwijk P, et al. Prognostic significance of ST segment shift early after resolution of ST elevation in patients with myocardial infarction treated with thrombolytic therapy: the GUSTO-I ST Segment Monitoring Substudy. J Am Coll Cardiol 1998; 31: 783–9

42. Syed MA, Borzak S, Asfour A, et al. Single lead ST segment recovery: a simple, reliable measure of successful fibrinolysis after acute myocardial infarction. Am Heart J 2004; 147: 275–80

43. Klootwijk P, Meij S, van Es GA, et al. Comparison of usefulness of computer assisted continuous 48-h 3-lead with 12-lead ECG ischaemia monitoring for detection and quantitation of ischaemia in patients with unstable angina. Eur Heart J 1997; 18: 931–40

44. Goldberg S, Greenspon AJ, Urban PL, et al. Reperfusion arrhythmia: a marker of restoration of antegrade flow during intracoronary thrombolysis for acute myocardial infarction. Am Heart J 1983; 105: 26–32

45. Gressin V, Louvard Y, Pezzano M, Lardoux H. Holter recording of ventricular arrhythmias during intravenous thrombolysis for acute myocardial infarction. Am J Cardiol 1992; 69: 152–9

46. Gressin V, Gorgels A, Louvard Y, Lardoux H, Bigelow R. ST segment normalization time and ventricular arrhythmias as electrocardiographic markers of reperfusion during intravenous thrombolysis for acute myocardial infarction. Am J Cardiol 1993; 71: 1436–9

47. Santoro GM, Valenti R, Buonamici P, et al. Relation between ST segment changes and myocardial perfusion evaluated by myocardial contrast echocardiography in patients with acute myocardial infarction treated with direct angioplasty. Am J Cardiol 1998; 82: 932–7

48. Ito H, Tomooka T, Sakai N, et al. Lack of myocardial perfusion immediately after successful thrombolysis. A predictor of poor recovery of left ventricular function in anterior myocardial infarction. Circulation 1992; 85: 1699–705

49. Antman EM, Anbe DT, Armstrong PW, et al. ACC/AHA guidelines for the management of patients with ST elevation myocardial infarction – executive summary. A report of the American College of Cardiology/American Heart Association Task Force on Practice Guidelines (Writing Committee to revise the 1999 guidelines for the management of patients with acute myocardial infarction). J Am Coll Cardiol 2004; 44: 671–719

50. Maas AC, Wyatt CM, Green CL, et al. Combining baseline clinical descriptors and real-time response to therapy: the incremental prognostic value of continuous ST segment monitoring in acute myocardial infarction. Am Heart J 2004; 147: 698–704

51. de Lemos JA, Morrow DA, Gibson CM, et al. Early noninvasive detection of failed epicardial reperfusion after fibrinolytic therapy. Am J Cardiol 2001; 88: 353–8

9

Rescue percutaneous coronary intervention in acute myocardial infarction

Omer Goktekin, Carlo Di Mario, Jun Tanigawa, Anthony Gershlick

DEFINITION

'Rescue' angioplasty is defined as the referral for urgent mechanical revascularization of a presumably occluded infarct-related artery (IRA) after failed intravenous thrombolysis. Rescue angioplasty must be distinguished from: (1) 'primary' angioplasty, i.e. a direct revascularization without preliminary administration of lytics; (2) 'facilitated' angioplasty, i.e. a planned immediate mechanical recanalization after intravenous thrombolytics or intravenous anti-platelet agents carried out irrespective of the results of the pharmacological treatment; (3) delayed elective angioplasty, i.e. a non-urgent mechanical intervention performed hours (or days) after thrombolytic therapy in the absence of new episodes of acute prolonged ischemia and ST segment elevation. 'Rescue' angioplasty requires a careful monitoring of the first 60–90 min and a prompt reaction to the lack of evidence of reperfusion. Every additional time period without reperfusion has adverse consequences by increasing the myocardial damage, especially in patients who present soon after symptom onset. An equally rapid referral is needed in cases of suspected reocclusion after initially successful thrombolysis, an event that may occur days after the initial infarction. In general the term 'rescue' percutaneous coronary intervention (PCI) refers to patients treated within 24 h from initial administration of lytics for the initial infarction. Urgent angioplasty days after an initially successful thrombolysis because of suspected reocclusion must be considered as primary angioplasty of a re-infarction.

INTRODUCTION

Intravenous thrombolysis remains the most frequently applied therapy for acute myocardial infarction (AMI) because of its widespread availability, but thrombolysis is not always able to achieve optimal reperfusion of the IRA. In the angiographic study of the Global Utilization of Streptokinase and Tissue Plasminogen Activator for Occluded Coronary Arteries (GUSTO-I) trial, the 90-min arterial patency rate, defined by the presence of TIMI grade 2 or 3 flow, was 54% in patients who received streptokinase, with only 29% of patients having TIMI grade 3 flow.[1] Administration of accelerated tissue plasminogen activators yielded superior early flow rates, but still restored TIMI 3 flow in only 54% of patients. Infarct artery patency is a powerful predictor of outcome in patients with AMI,[2] with several trials highlighting the relation between flow restoration in the IRA at 90 min after initiation of thrombolytic therapy and subsequent mortality.[3,4] In a pooled analysis of five studies of 3969 patients that examined the relationship between early TIMI grade and mortality after AMI, overall mortality was 8.8% for TIMI grade 0/1, 7.0% for grade 2 and 3.7% for perfusion TIMI grade 3.[5] Acute and convalescent ejection fraction, regional wall motion, peak enzyme levels and risk of heart failure were all better in patients achieving TIMI perfusion grade 3 compared to grade 2 or lower.

IDENTIFICATION OF CANDIDATES FOR RESCUE ANGIOPLASTY

Failure of initial reperfusion

Detection of patients with failed thrombolysis at an early stage is crucial, to allow consideration of alternative reperfusion therapy before irreversible myocardial necrosis occurs. However, identification of patients with failed thrombolysis is problematic. Failure of thrombolysis may be suggested by severe, persistent, unchanged or worsened chest pain after administration of lytics. Anxiety, fear, pericardial pain and the confounding effect of analgesics make this parameter unreliable. Furthermore, pain is not involved in the 15–20% of patients with silent myocardial infarction (MI). Rapid resolution of chest pain is associated with increased probability of a patent IRA[6–8] and TIMI grade 3 flow (84%).[9] Persistent chest pain is not sufficient to guide decisions about rescue angioplasty because 60% of the patients with unchanged or worsened chest pain with ST segment resolution have a patent IRA.[6] ECG changes and in particular ST segment resolution determined at the time when lytics are likely to achieve the greatest reperfusion (60–90 min) are more reliable and objective parameters. Although the presence of early resolution of ST segment elevation is indicative of a patent IRA, an incomplete ST segment resolution ($\leq$50% in the lead with maximal ST segment elevation) remains an unspecific predictor of IRA occlusion (still associated with 63% epicardial patency, with some of the remaining cases possibly reflecting irreversible myocardial tissue damage).[6,10,11] Biochemical markers, particularly CK-MB and troponin I or T, are potentially useful non-invasive markers of reperfusion. A rapid increase in the serum concentration of cardiac biomarkers over the first 60–90 min after fibrinolysis can help to identify patients who have achieved successful reperfusion.[7,12] Although myoglobin appears to be superior to CK-MB and troponin for this purpose,[13] it has the same limitations of the measurement of ST. While a rapid increase in myoglobin is highly predictive of a patent IRA, the absence of rapid myoglobin 'washout' has a poor positive predictive value for the presence of an occluded IRA.[12,13] Furthermore, the blood sample must be swiftly processed and analyzed, a goal difficult to achieve out of hours and in small hospitals.

The TIMI 14 trial investigators proposed a strategy using a combination of electrocardiography, chest pain and serum markers to identify patients with angiographic evidence of failed thrombolysis (TIMI flow grade < 3) who would then be candidates for rescue PCI.[11] Three criteria were used: (1) < 50% ST resolution at 90 min; (2) persistence of chest pain; and (3) reduced washout of myoglobin (ratio of 60-min to baseline myoglobin levels of < 4). Patients who met any individual criterion were more likely to have less than TIMI 3 flow or an occluded infarct-related artery (TIMI 0/1 flow) than those who did not meet the criterion ($p < 0.005$ for each). When the three criteria were used together ($n = 169$), patients who satisfied 0 ($n = 29$), 1 ($n = 68$), 2 ($n = 51$), or 3 ($n = 21$) of the criteria had a 17%, 24%, 35% and 76% probability of failing to achieve TIMI 3 flow ($p < 0.0001$) and a 0%, 6%, 18% and 57% probability of a persistently occluded IRA, respectively ($p < 0.0001$). Patients who satisfied all three non-invasive criteria had a 70% probability of achieving less than TIMI grade 3 flow, a 50% probability of an occluded IRA and a 10-fold increase in the risk for 30-day mortality versus those with 0 or 1 criteria present. Patients meeting two of the three criteria have an intermediate probability of fibrinolytic failure.[14]

Other non-invasive methods such as transthoracic echocardiography, contrast echocardiography, magnetic resonance imaging and nuclear imaging with ^{99m}Tc-labeled sestamibi can also be used to determine IRA patency after thrombolysis. It has been shown that the demonstration of a restored flow in the infarct-related artery by using transthoracic echocardiography is feasible soon after thrombolysis (15 min to 6 h).[15] Lee et al. performed transthoracic echocardiography in 46 consecutive patients with a first anterior AMI in the acute phase before emergency coronary intervention. The presence of antegrade distal left anterior descending artery flow and its diastolic peak velocity were evaluated by color and pulsed Doppler and compared with TIMI grades by subsequent coronary angiography performed 29 ± 12 min later. They found that transthoracic echocardiography enabled non-invasive differentiation of TIMI 3 from TIMI ≤ 2 coronary reperfusion in patients with AMI in the acute phase before emergency coronary angioplasty.[16] Contrast echocardiography and other techniques of myocardial tissue imaging show microvascular myocardial perfusion rather than epicardial patency. Although a patent epicardial coronary artery is a prerequisite for successful reperfusion, the presence of TIMI-3 flow is not a guarantee for successful reperfusion at the microvascular level. Myocardial contrast echocardiography showed that one-fourth to one-third of patients showed lack of microvascular flow (no-reflow) despite a fully patent coronary artery.[17] Wackers et al. evaluated the efficacy of technetium-99m isonitrile myocardial perfusion scintigraphy to assess the success of thrombolytic therapy.[18] Twenty-three patients underwent technetium-99m isonitrile myocardial perfusion scintigraphy before thrombolytic therapy. Repeat imaging was performed 18–48 h later and at 6–14 days after the onset of myocardial infarction to visualize the ultimate extent of infarction. Patients with a patent IRA had a significantly greater decrease in defect size than did patients with persistent coronary occlusion ($-51 \pm 38\%$ vs. $-1 \pm 26\%$, $p = 0.0001$). The need of a baseline examination and the half-life of the radioisotope, besides the time and complexity of this approach, make it unlikely that the magnitude of the 'salvage index', the difference between poST and pre-image, is used as an immediate indicator of efficacy of lytics.

Magnetic resonance (MR) and 64-multislice computed tomography (MS-CT) offer the possibility of direct non-invasive coronary imaging. In a study of Hundley et al.[19] in 18 patients, proximal, middle and distal segments of infarct arteries were classified as having antegrade, collateral, or no flow. The infarct artery was the left anterior descending in ten patients, the right coronary artery in seven, and the circumflex in one. When compared with the results of contrast angiography, MR imaging correctly identified the presence or absence of antegrade flow in the infarct artery of all 18 patients. Similar or better results may be expected with 64 MS-CT, although screening of patients with suspected thoracic pain is the only practical acute cardiac indication proposed and tested for this novel technique so far.

Reocclusion after successful thrombolysis

Failure to reperfuse is the main trigger for rescue PCI but an equally adverse condition that is more difficult to diagnose promptly and treat is recurrent occlusion of the IRA. Reocclusion of the IRA after successful thrombolytic therapy occurs in 5–30% of patients during the in-hospital period.[20] The combination of a high-grade thrombus containing lesion, platelet activation induced by most lytics and the limited protection offered by heparin and aspirin explain the high frequency of this event. Thrombotic coronary occlusion can be manifested by ST segment re-elevation, recurrent chest pain, hemodynamic deterioration or by a second peak of cardiac enzymes. However, 78% of reocclusions are not associated with clinically overt symptoms or apparent reinfarction.[21] Clinical reinfarction has been documented in only 4% of patients in the first week of hospital stay.[22] Reinfarction rate is higher if the patient is female, older than 70 years, has had a previous MI or a history of hypertension.[23] The 2004 ACC/AHA Task Force issued specific guidelines for the diagnosis of reinfarction after an acute MI.[24] Within the first 18 h of the initial MI, a recurrent elevation in cardiac biomarkers alone is not sufficient to diagnose reinfarction, but should be accompanied by recurrent ST segment elevation or recurrent chest pain and/or hemodynamic deterioration. After the first 18 h from the initial MI, a rise of troponin or CK-MB of at least 50% from the previous measurement and at least one additional clinical criterion are sufficient for the diagnosis to be made.

The prognostic significance of recurrent ST segment changes after initial normalization in ST elevation MI patients treated with thrombolysis has been studied in the GUSTO-I Segment Monitoring Substudy.[25] Of 734 patients, 243 (33%) had a new ST segment shift (elevation or depression). The 30-day mortality rate in patients with an ST shift was 7.8%, significantly higher than in patients without an ST segment shift (2.25%, $p = 0.001$). A similar difference was observed for the 1-year mortality rate (10.3% vs. 5.7%, $p = 0.02$). In a pooled analysis of 20 101 patients from TIMI 4, 9 and 10B and InTIME-I trials ($n = 836$), in-hospital reinfarction occurred in 4.2% of patients with significant ST segment abnormalities.[23] Recurrent

MI in hospital was associated with increased 30-day mortality (16.4% vs. 6.2%, $p < 0.001$), with a persistent significant difference up to 2 years.

RESCUE PCI FOR FAILED THROMBOLYSIS AND REOCCLUSION

Several registries but very few randomized studies have evaluated the role of rescue angioplasty after failed thrombolysis or for early reocclusion of an IRA. Moreover, most of these studies were performed before the use of stenting or glycoprotein IIb/IIIa inhibitors became common practice. For this reason the applicability of some of these studies is limited.

Non-randomized and observational studies

Rescue PCI was evaluated first in the 1980s in non-randomized studies, and success rates of these first pioneer experiences of rescue angioplasty were lower than the success rate reported for primary PCI.[26–28] An observational report by Abbottsmith *et al.* suggested no difference in mortality between patients failing thrombolytic therapy who were treated with rescue angioplasty compared to those treated conservatively.[28] At hospital discharge, mortality in the rescue group was 9.9% versus 6.9% in the medical group. Mortality in patients with failed rescue angioplasty was significantly greater than in those with an angiographically successful outcome (39% vs. 6%, $p < 0.05$). A pooled analysis by Ellis *et al.* confirmed a high overall mortality rate (10.6%) and no improvement in left ventricular function in the week after rescue PCI. They also reported that reocclusion after successful rescue PCI occurred in up to 29% of patients.[29]

The role of rescue PCI after failure of thrombolytic therapy was also evaluated retrospectively in subset analyses of the TIMI trials. While the first TIMI trials (TIMI 1, 2 and 4) suggested that routine use of rescue PCI after thrombolytic failure does not offer significant benefit over medical therapy, the later TIMI 10B and TIMI 14 trials suggested improved outcome after angioplasty, probably reflecting the improved PCI technique and concomitant pharmacological treatment. The outcome of 100 consecutive patients with no rescue PCI in the TIMI I trial was compared with the outcome observed in 33 consecutive patients undergoing rescue PCI in the TIMI II trial. Rescue PCI was successful in 82% and the mortality rate at 21 days was 12% in the rescue group and 7% in the no-rescue group (NS).[30] Failure to achieve reperfusion after rescue angioplasty was again associated with a mortality as high as 33%. Reinfarction occurred in 6% of the patients in the rescue group. Mean left ventricular ejection fraction at 21 days was similar in the rescue and no-rescue group (51 ± 13% vs. 48 ± 12%, respectively (NS)). The results of this analysis suggest that routine rescue PCI does not significantly influence outcome compared with medical therapy. However, this study was not randomized, had a duration of follow-up of only 21 days and the indication for rescue PCI was angiographically documented persistent occlusion at 90 min and not residual or recurrent ischemia or hemodynamic instability. Therefore, it is possible that this group represented a low-risk population.

In the TIMI 4 trial the angiographic and clinical outcomes of patients with a patent artery 90 min after thrombolysis were compared with the outcome of patients with an occluded artery either treated with PCI or left untreated.[31] In-hospital adverse outcome (death, recurrent AMI, severe congestive heart failure, cardiogenic shock or an ejection fraction of < 40%) occurred in 35% of patients who underwent rescue PCI (successes and failures combined) vs. 23% in patients with a patent IRA after thrombolysis ($p = 0.07$).

Rescue PCI was also assessed in more recent TIMI trials such as TIMI 10B and 14. A total of 1938 patients from the TIMI 10B and 14 trials were evaluated.[32] All patients underwent angiography 90 min after thrombolysis, and from 372 patients with TIMI grade 0 or 1, 293 underwent, at the discretion of the investigator, immediate rescue PCI; 55 patients had no PCI and 22 delayed PCI. There was a significantly lower 30-day mortality among patients who underwent immediate rescue PCI than among those who did not (6% vs. 17%, $p = 0.01$). Longer follow-up at 2 years from the TIMI 10B trial suggested a significant mortality benefit in the 80% of patients who underwent rescue PCI (13% vs. 27%, hazard ratio 0.34 after adjusting for the use of stents).

Table 9.1 Early randomized trials of rescue percutaneous coronary intervention in patients with occluded infarct-related arteries

	Belenkie et al.	RESCUE	Combined
No. of patients	28	151	368
Anterior MI (%)	53.6	100.0	
In-hospital or 30-day death (%)			
PTCA group	6.3	5.1	8.5
Medical group (%)	33.3	9.6	12.2
In-hospital or 30-day repeat MI (%)			
PTCA group	—	—	4.3
Medical group	—	—	11.3
30-day CHF (%)			
PTCA group	—	1.3	3.8
Medical group	—	7.0	11.7*
Re-intervention 6 months (%)			
PTCA group	—	16.6	
Medical group	—	23.3	

MI, myocardial infarction; PTCA, percutaneous transluminal coronary angioplasty; CHF, congestive heart failure
*$p \leq 0.05$ vs. conservative group

Randomized trials

To date four small and two larger randomized controlled trials have been conducted to determine whether or not rescue PCI is beneficial in patients with evidence of failed thrombolysis or early reocclusion after thrombolysis (Table 9.1).

Belenkie et al. randomly assigned 28 patients with a persistently occluded IRA after thrombolytic therapy to either PCI ($n = 16$) or conservative treatment ($n = 12$). There was a non-significant trend for a lower in-hospital mortality rate in the rescue PCI group (6.3% compared with 33.3%, $p = 0.13$).[33]

The RESCUE I (Randomized Evaluation of Salvage Angioplasty with Combined Utilization of Endpoints) study is the first reasonably large trial that has specifically addressed rescue percutaneous transluminal coronary angioplasty (PTCA).[32] The RESCUE I study included 151 patients with first anterior myocardial infarction who were treated with thrombolytic therapy and were shown to have an occluded IRA (TIMI flow 0 or 1) within 8 h of pain onset. These patients were randomly assigned to undergo rescue PCI ($n = 78$) or conservative medical management ($n = 73$). The RESCUE I trial investigators reported a technical success rate of 92.3% (defined as final TIMI flow grade ≥ 2 and residual stenosis < 50%), higher than the patency reported in previous series. The study reported no difference in the primary study endpoint of resting left ventricular ejection fraction at 30 days but the exercise ejection fraction at 30 days was higher in the rescue PCI group (43% vs. 38%, $p = 0.04$). There were also trends toward lower 30-day mortality (5.1% compared with 9.6%, $p = 0.18$) and less frequent development of heart failure (1.3% compared with 7.0%, $p = 0.11$) in the rescue PCI group. A statistically significant benefit was reported in the rescue PCI group for the combined outcome of death or severe congestive heart failure at 30 days (6.4% vs. 16.6%; $p < 0.05$). These differences were still present at 1-year follow-up. Furthermore, it should be noted that the benefits of rescue PCI were most likely to be underestimated by this study as a result of the exclusion of patients with previous MI by protocol and the investigator bias to undertake PCI (and therefore not to randomize) 134 other high-risk patients with left anterior descending occlusion. Patients who were seen particularly early (< 3 h from chest pain onset) after MI (perhaps those most likely to benefit) also tended not to be included in this study. A meta-analysis of the pooled data on 1-year follow-up from RESCUE I and the study of Belenkie et al. revealed a clear-cut and statistically significant survival advantage for patients randomly assigned to rescue PCI.[34,35]

There are also published trials of delayed angioplasty in patients with partially occluded (TIMI 2 flow) vessels following thrombolytic therapy (Table 9.2). The first of these was the Thrombolysis and Angioplasty in Myocardial Infarction (TAMI) I study, performed during 1985 and 1986: angioplasty was successfully performed in 79% of patients.[36] Among patients with TIMI 2 flow grade there were no differences of in-hospital death or congestive heart failure in the angioplasty versus medical therapy arms (6.1 vs. 1.7%, $p = 0.25$ and 18.4 vs. 23.7%, $p = 0.50$). However, there was a trend, particularly when angioplasty was performed within 5 h of chest pain onset, that left ventricular ejection fraction (LVEF) might be improved (increment from

Table 9.2 Randomized trials of rescue pecutaneous coronary intervention (PCI) in patients with TIMI grade 2 flow

| | TAMI 1 | | RESCUE II | |
	PCI	Conservative	PCI	Conservative
No. of patients	49	59	14	15
Anterior MI (%)	41	42	79*	40
LVEF (%)	51 ± 12	54 ± 10	44 ± 10	45 ± 9
Outcomes (30-day)				
mortality (%)	6.1	1.7	7.1	0.0
LVEF (%)	52 ± 11	53 ± 12	53 ± 10	41 ± 10
Recurrent MI/ischemia (%)	–/5	–/16*	0/21.4	0/46.7
One year mortality (%)	8.2	3.4	7.1	6.7

MI, myocardial infarction; LVEF, left ventricular ejection fraction

*$p \leq 0.05$ vs. conservative group

baseline to 7/10-day follow-up: 3.3 ± 8.0 vs. 1.4 ± 8.1, $p = 02$). The RESCUE II trial was designed to test the hypothesis that, in patients with TIMI 2 flow in the IRA following thrombolysis, coronary intervention would improve clinical outcomes compared with conservative medical therapy.[37] Although only 29 patients could be randomized, results at 30 days and 12 months showed that there was less elective or urgent revascularization in the angioplasty group. At 12 months, the incidences of death, repeat MI, coronary artery bypass grafting, and need for further PTCA were 7.1%, 0.0%, 7.1% and 21.4% in the PTCA group, respectively, and 6.7%, 0.0%, 0.0% and 46.7% in the conservative group. In the eight patients in the PTCA group with LVEF assessed at 6 months, the mean increase was 9 ± 13%, compared with 4 ± 5% in the seven patients in the conservative group ($p = 0.027$).

Using data from the GUSTO-1 angiographic substudy, Ross et al. compared the clinical and angiographic outcomes of 198 patients undergoing rescue PTCA, 266 patients with failed thrombolysis managed conservatively and 1058 patients with successful thrombolysis.[38] Rescue angioplasty did not increase catheterization laboratory or poST procedural complication rates. Multivariate analysis identified severe heart failure to be the only determinant of a failed rescue attempt. Successful rescue PCI was associated with a better left ventricular function and lower 30-day mortality when compared to the outcome in patients with closed IRAs managed conservatively. The outcome was, however, still less favorable than in patients in whom thrombolytic therapy was initially successful. The mortality rate after a failed rescue attempt was 30.4%. It should be noted that five of the seven patients who died after failed rescue PTCA were in cardiogenic shock before the procedure.

All the above data reflect treatment in patients prior to the routine use of intracoronary stenting and modern anti-platelet therapy which are known to improve clinical outcomes. However, two recent major randomized studies have evaluated the success rate and outcome of rescue PCI in the setting of contemporary practice.

MERLIN trial

The Middlesbrough Early Revascularization to Limit Infarction (MERLIN) trial included 307 patients with ST elevation MI who were treated with streptokinase and in whom an ECG obtained after 60 min showed incomplete ST segment resolution (< 50% improvement from presentation).[39] Ongoing chest pain at the time of arrival in the catheterization laboratory was not a requirement for enrollment. Patients were randomly assigned to transfer for rescue PCI versus medical therapy. In the rescue PCI arm, TIMI 3 flow in the IRA was achieved in 130 patients (85%). Thirty-day all-cause mortality was similar in the rescue and conservative groups (9.8% vs. 11%, $p = 0.7$). The composite secondary endpoint of death/re-infarction/-stroke/subsequent revascularization/heart failure occurred less commonly in the rescue PCI arm (37.3% vs. 50%, $p = 0.02$) due to reduction in ischemia-driven revascularization (6.5% vs. 20.1%). However, stroke and bleeding requiring transfusion were more common in patients undergoing rescue PCI (4.6% vs. 0.6%, $p = 0.03$ and 11.1% vs. 1.3%, $p < 0.001$). Left ventricular function at 30 days was the same in the two groups. It should be noted that, because the trial was underpowered (300 patients) to detect a difference in the primary endpoint (mortality), the negative conclusion of the trial (similar mortality in the two groups) could simply be a type II error. Other limitations of the MERLIN trial include very early randomization after thrombolysis and a high prevalence of inferior MI.[40]

REACT

The REACT (REscue Angioplasty vs. Conservative treatment or repeat Thrombolysis) was a multicenter, randomized, parallel group study conducted between 2000 and 2004. A total of 435 patients were randomized in 35 centers, 19 of which had on-site angiographic facilities. The trial set out to compare three treatment options in patients with failed thrombolysis: (1) repeat administration of lytics ('RESCUE-Lysis'); (2) conservative therapy (ongoing treatment with heparin only); and (3) 'RESCUE-PCI'.[41] Patients aged between 21 and 85 years were eligible for inclusion in the trial if, despite receiving any licensed thrombolytics for AMI within 6 h of onset of chest pain, they failed to reperfuse as judged by failure to achieve > 50% resolution in the lead with previous maximal ST segment elevation 90 min after the lytics. The primary endpoint was the composite of major adverse cardiac and cerebrovascular events (MACCE) of all deaths, re-AMI, cerebrovascular event (CVA) or severe heart failure at 6 months.

Twelve patients (15.3%) in the rescue-PCI treatment arm met at least one endpoint within 6 months, compared to 44 (31.0%) in the rescue-lysis group and 42 (29.8%) in the conservative group (overall $p = 0.003$). The event-free survival curves (Kaplan–Meier) for all treatment groups are presented in Figure 9.1. Of the rescue-PCI arm 84.6% (95% CI 78.7–90.5%) were event-free at 6 months, compared to 70.1% (95% CI 62.5–77.7%) of the conservative group and 68.7% (95% CI 61.1–76.4%) of the rescue-lysis group (overall $p = 0.004$). The event rates displayed in a predetermined hierarchical ranking are shown in Table 9.3. Bleeding events were captured during the index admission via clinical and hematology assessments at various time-points up to discharge. There were no significant differences between the

Figure 9.1   Time to first event at 6 months (*n* = 427). R-PCI, rescue percutaneous coronary intervention; C, conservative treatment; R-Lysis, rescue lysis.

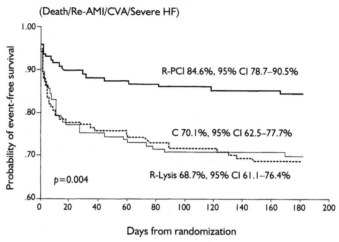

Treatment	No. of event-free subjects Timepoints (days)								
Group	20	40	60	80	100	120	140	160	180
R-Lysis	110	106	105	101	99	99	96	95	93
C	109	104	102	99	98	97	96	95	93
R-PCI	129	127	124	122	120	118	117	116	115

Table 9.3   REACT trial: no. of subjects with endpoint events within 6 months

	Re-lysis (n = 142)	Conservation (n = 141)	R-PCI (n = 144)	Overall p value
Primary endpoint events: predetermined hierarchical analysis				
Death	18 (12.7%)	18 (12.8%)	9 (6.3%)	p = 0.120
(cardiac)	15 (10.6%)	14 (9.9%)	8 (5.6%)	p = 0.261
Re-AMI	15 (10.6%)	12 (8.5%)	3 (2.1%)	p = 0.007
CVA	1 (0.7%)	1 (0.7%)	3 (2.1%)	p = 0.626
Severe HF	10 (7.0%)	11 (7.8%)	7 (4.9%)	p = 0.581
Composite	44 (31%)	42 (29.8%)	22 (15.3%)	p = 0.003
Secondary endpoint: bleeding events				
Major bleed				
↓Hb + over bleed	7 (4.9%) (1 death)	3 (2.1%) (1 death)	27 (18.7%)	p = 0.0001
↓Hb − over bleed	12 (8.5%)	12 (8.5%)	12 (8.3%)	p = 0.151
Over bleed alone	5 (3.5%) (4 deaths)	3 (2.1%) (2 deaths)	0 (0.0%)	p = 0.055
Minor bleed				
Over bleed	5 (3.5%)	5 (3.5%)	8 (5.6%)	p = 0.617
No over bleed	22 (15.5%)	22 (15.6%)	16 (11.1%)	p = 0.459
Secondary endpoint: revascularization				
PCI/CABG	33 (23.2%)	29 (20.6%)	19 (13.2%)	p = 0.080

Re-lysis, repeat thrombolytics; R-PCI, rescue percutaneous coronary intervention; Re-AMI, re-acute myocardial infarction; CVA, cardiovascular accident; HF, heart failure; CABG, coronary artery bypass graft groups with respect to mortality or minor bleeding events. A tendency towards higher fatal bleeding was noted in both the conservative and repeat thrombolytic arms, but no firm conclusions can be drawn given the small number of events that occurred.

At 6 months freedom from re-vascularization, a predetermined secondary endpoint, was 86.7% in the rescue-PCI group (95% CI 81.1–92.3%) compared to 79.3% in the conservative group (95% CI 72.6–86.0%) and 76.5% in the rescue group (95% CI 69.5–83.5%) (overall $p = 0.076$).

REACT was the first study to compare three therapeutic options currently utilized following failed thrombolysis. It has clearly demonstrated that a mechanical intervention using rescue percutaneous coronary angioplasty is superior to either conservative care or administering repeat thrombolytics, which had no benefit.

ADJUVANT PHARMALOGICAL THERAPY DURING RESCUE PCI

Glycoprotein IIb/IIIa inhibitors

The rationale for the use of GPIIb/IIIa inhibitors in rescue PCI is based on their potent anti-platelet effect, which may be useful after failed thrombolysis. In fact, thrombolysis promotes platelet aggregation due to the release of thrombin from the fibrin network of the thrombus and the production of the proaggregatory fibrin degradation products. Thus, whether or not a successful mechanical resolution has been achieved, a mechanical intervention such as angioplasty soon after lytics is conducted in a phase of enhanced platelet activation, which may lead to embolization or new occlusion.

Abciximab is a safe adjunctive therapy for patients receiving primary PCI, and in a pooled analysis of the trials RAPPORT, CADILLAC, ISAR-2, ADMIRAL and ACE there was a 46% reduction in death or reinfarction, or target vessel revascularization, a 34% reduction in death or reinfarction, and a (non-significant) 26% reduction in death at 1 month in the abciximab group.[42] The safety of glycoprotein IIb/IIIa inhibitors in the setting of rescue or urgent PCI after full-dose thrombolytic therapy remains, however, unclear. Very few studies have described the use of glycoprotein IIb/IIIa inhibitors during rescue PCI. Three small retrospective evaluations of glycoprotein IIb/IIIa inhibitors used during rescue angioplasty point toward a moderate increase in risk of major bleeding compared with standard therapy.[43–45] The largest study examining the efficacy and complications of glycoprotein IIb/IIIa inhibition during rescue PCI after full-dose fibrinolysis is the Global Use of Strategies to Open Occluded Coronary Arteries (GUSTO) III trial.[46] Of the 15 059 patients enrolled, 393 patients underwent PCI a median of 3.5 h after thrombolysis and had complete procedural data. When compared, the 30-day mortality in patients who received abciximab ($n = 83$) and in patients who did not ($n = 309$) tended to be lower with abciximab (3.6% vs. 9.7%, $p = 0.07$). Severe bleeding, however, occurred in 4% of patients in the abciximab group and 1% of patients in the standard therapy group (3.6% vs. 1.0%, $p = 0.08$).

The sub-analysis of the GUSTO V trial also showed benefit of abciximab in rescue PCI: 16 588 patients in the first 6 h of evolving ST segment elevation myocardial infarction were randomly assigned to standard-dose reteplase ($n = 8260$) or half-dose reteplase and full-dose abciximab ($n = 8328$).[47] The use of percutaneous coronary intervention was discouraged by protocol and its utilization within 6 h was 8.6% in the reteplase group versus 5.6% in the reteplase–abciximab group (0.64 (0.56–0.72), $p < 0.0001$), suggesting improved early patency or reduced early reocclusion with abciximab on board. All-cause mortality at 30 days in the early PCI group was 6.6% for the reteplase group ($n = 441$), compared with 3.0% for the combined reteplase and abciximab group ($n = 266$), $p < 0.01$.

Another small randomized study, in patients receiving abciximab ($n = 44$) or placebo ($n = 45$) during rescue PCI showed a significant improvement of echocardiographic left ventricular motion at 30-day follow-up (0.28 vs. 0.12, $p < 0.001$). In the abciximab group, a significant reduction in major adverse cardiac events (death, MI, failure) was observed at 6-month follow-up (11% vs. 38%, $p = 0.004$). The incidence of major, moderate and minor bleeding was similar in the two groups (20% vs. 16%).[48]

Until further data become available, the decision regarding the use of glycoprotein IIb/IIIa inhibition during rescue PCI should be made on a case-by-case basis weighing the magnitude of potential benefits against bleeding risk. Factors to be considered are the type of lytics used (possibly avoid after streptokinase), time after end of lytic infusion (more caution in the first 1–3 h after lytics), age and risk factors for bleeding (great caution in > 75-year-old patients, especially if hypertensive).

Clopidogrel

Adding the anti-platelet agent clopidogrel to standard reperfusion therapy for patients with ST elevation myocardial infarction significantly reduces their rate of blocked culprit coronary artery, death or recurrent MI by the time of angiography. In the Clopidogrel as Adjunctive Reperfusion Therapy (CLARITY) Thrombolysis In Myocardial Infarction (TIMI) 28 trial, 3491 ST elevation MI patients undergoing fibrinolysis were randomized to clopidogrel, given as a loading dose of 300 mg, followed by 75 mg a day or placebo for an average of 4 days, until angiography.[49] Standard fibrinolytic agents and anticoagulants were used and all patients received aspirin. The patients underwent angiographic assessment 2–8 days after starting study medication. Patients who received clopidogrel had a significantly lower rate of a blocked culprit coronary artery, death or recurrent MI than control patients (15% in the clopidogrel group vs. 21.7% in the control group, $p < 0.000001$). This benefit held regardless of age, gender, type of fibrinolytic or type of heparin. By 30 days, patients treated with clopidogrel had a lower rate of death due to cardiovascular causes, recurrent MI, or recurrent ischemia leading to the need for urgent revascularization (11.6% in the clopidogrel group vs. 14.1% in the control group, $p = 0.03$). As no increased risk of bleeding was observed in this study, before shipping the patients for rescue PCI clopidogrel should be routinely used as currently advised in other acute (non-ST elevation MI) or elective patients undergoing PCI.[50,51]

TECHNICAL RECOMMENDATIONS FOR RESCUE PCI

Rescue PCI has a lower success and higher reocclusion rate compared with primary PCI. Even before the elective stenting era, the availability of stents for bail-out increased the success rate of rescue PCI up to 88–95%.[38,52] The extensive use of stents in current clinical practice has further improved the success rate and clinical outcome. Several observational studies have demonstrated that a stent can be safely deployed in the thrombogenic substrate of failed thrombolysis and is associated with improved angiographic and clinical results compared with rescue balloon angioplasty.[53–55] Data from the Stent or Percutaneous Transluminal Coronary Angioplasty for Occluded Coronary Arteries in Patients With Acute Myocardial Infarction (STOPAMI) investigators indicate that stenting after failed thrombolysis is associated with greater myocardial salvage than balloon angioplasty alone.[56] Overall these studies suggest that patients with failed thrombolysis should undergo rescue stenting.

The use of intra-aortic balloon counterpulsation (IABP) has also been suggested to improve outcome in rescue PCI. The Randomized IABP Study Group randomly assigned 182 patients sent for emergency cardiac catheterization within 24 h of acute myocardial infarction, including 51 patients undergoing rescue PTCA, to a prolonged (48 h) treatment with IABP or standard care.[57] After angiography in the IABP group significant reductions were noted for the combined endpoint of death, stroke and recurrent ischemic events (13% vs. 24% with standard therapy, $p = 0.04$), and for reocclusion (8% vs. 21% with standard therapy, $p < 0.03$). Only one study specifically addressed the use of IABP in the setting of rescue PCI. Ishihara and associates[58] non-randomly assigned the first 20 consecutive patients with anterior myocardial infarction who underwent rescue PCI to standard care and the following 40 patients with similar characteristics to the use of IABP. The patients treated with IABP had significantly lower reocclusion rates (2.5% compared with 25.0%; $p < 0.05$), better predischarge ejection fraction (6.8% increase vs. 2.0% decrease; $p < 0.05$), and a non-significant trend toward decreased mortality (5.0% vs. 20.0%; $p > 0.05$). These results suggest that IABP may be helpful in patients undergoing rescue PCI.

Atheromatous and thrombotic embolization during PCI in AMI is common and may result in microcirculatory dysfunction. Its prevention is imperative to improve reperfusion success and reduce infarct size. Because failure of thrombolysis is associated with an increased thrombus burden,[59] potentially the use of thrombectomy can be particularly beneficial in the setting of rescue PCI. Several devices that can mechanically aspirate thrombus are available, including the transluminal extraction catheter (TEC), the AngioJet and the X-Sizer. Recently, Lee et al. evaluated the safety and feasibility of X-Sizer-assisted rescue PCI ($n = 15$) after failed thrombolysis using the success rate and clinical outcome after X-Sizer-assisted primary PCI for comparison ($n = 80$).[60] Angiographic success rate was achieved in 100% in the rescue PCI group and 96% in the primary PCI group. At 30-day and 6-month follow-up, mortality rate, major acute coronary event and angina rates were similar between the rescue group and the primary group.

A number of small single-center experiences have demonstrated retrieval of macroscopic atherothrombotic debris in 70–90% of patients with AMI undergoing primary or rescue PCI with distal protection, with improved angiographic outcomes, ST segment resolution and/or myocardial recovery compared with historical controls.[61–63] Stone and colleagues[64] reported the results of the Enhanced Myocardial Efficacy and Removal by Aspiration of Liberated Debris (EMERALD) randomized trial, which was designed to assess the efficacy of protection of the coronary microcirculation by use of balloon occlusion and an aspiration protection device (Guardwire Plus, Medtronic, USA) in patients with AMI undergoing primary and rescue PCI ($n = 45$). Among the patients assigned to distal protection, successful deployment of a distal occlusion balloon and subsequent aspiration was performed in 97% (242/251), with all dilatations fully protected in 79%. Despite this high device success rate and the presence of visible debris in 73% of cases, the use of protection devices was not associated with increased complete ST resolution (63.3% vs. 61.9% in the control group, $p = 0.78$), or reduced left ventricular infarct size (12.0% vs. 9.5% in the control group, $p = 0.15$) or improved 6-month clinical outcome (10.0% vs. 11.0% in the control group, $p = 0.6$). Also, no advantages with distal protection were seen in the rescue PCI sub-group.

The most powerful predictors of vascular and bleeding complications occurring at the femoral puncture site are obesity, hypertension and rescue PCI. Access site complications can represent a significant complication in terms of morbidity, duration of hospitalization and procedural costs. To minimize the vascular access complications, extra precautions are needed for sheath removal and hemostasis control in rescue PCI. In selected patients the use of closure devices including collagen plug devices or percutaneous suture closure devices may reduce vascular complications. In our practice we routinely use the closure device in rescue PCI unless the femoral vessels are very small, diffusely narrowed and heavily calcified. Both after closure device and manual compression a prolonged use of bed rest and of low-pressure compression with a Femostop reduces the frequent oozing and blood infiltration.

To avoid the vascular access complications almost completely a transradial approach is highly recommended in rescue PCI.[65] The radial approach practically eliminates the risk of access-site large hemorrhage as this small superficial vessel is a site where bleeding is very easy to control (wrist bands can be used for many hours, with great patient comfort, waiting for the end of the effect of lytics). With sufficient experience and rare exceptions, achievement of patency of the culprit vessel in AMI is not delayed with the transradial approach compared to the transfemoral route in rescue PCI. The radial approach, however, cannot be used for intra-aortic balloon pump insertion.

CONCLUSION

Even in countries with high socioeconomic standards objective organization problems limit the use of primary PCI to areas sufficiently close to interventional centers with 40–50% of patients with AMI still treated with PCI.

Patients with ongoing chest pain and/or hemodynamic compromise, but also asymptomatic patients with persistent > 50% ST segment elevation 60–90 min after lytic therapy, should undergo emergency angiography. Many other complex techniques have been proposed but, in reality, as the decision to refer to rescue angioplasty must be taken in a district hospital where none or few of these techniques are available, especially after hours, ECG and chest pain remain the only criteria of practical help. Obviously there might be exceptions with particularly efficient analysis laboratories providing results for myoglobin within minutes or accomplished echocardiography operators able to measure flow directly not only in the LAD, but the principle should be that, unless concordant evidence confirms reperfusion at 60–90 min, one should never take the risk not to ascertain a persistent failure of thrombolysis, suggesting a liberal policy of immediate transfer to a larger PCI hospital. The reorganization of the ambulance service to offer optimal treatment to patients with AMI should include immediate availability of dedicated equipped cars for rescue transfers, with an emergency code bypassing the routine slow pace of interhospital transfers.

The creation of dedicated equipped ambulance services has paradoxically increased the use of lytics in the form of prehospital thrombolysis. Although there is no clear evidence that immediate lysis in the ambulance is superior to primary angioplasty, necessarily performed after 60–120-min delay, both approaches are possibly valid if attention is paid to a prompt referral to rescue PCI in case of failure of thrombolytics. Ongoing trials of immediate vs. rescue or delayed elective angioplasty after lytics may clarify the best treatment option. At present, we suggest an extended indication to transfer. Even in patients who already achieved TIMI 3 flow, angiography is nevertheless required after ST elevation MI treated with thrombolysis and most of the arteries with a diameter of stenosis of > 50% will require PCI irrespective of TIMI flow. Stenting should be offered to all patients. The negative results of the only randomized trial with distal protection devices suggest limiting their use to the presence of gross thrombotic burden. Similarly, IABP during or after rescue should be reserved to patients with hypotension not related to fluid deprivation or progressive hemodynamic compromise. A radial approach should be offered to all patients with rescue angioplasty. Prolonged compression and closure devices may help in 'femoral only' centers. All patients should arrive at the angioplasty center preloaded with clopidogrel. For recanalization of complex lesions and persistent occlusions, abciximab should be considered and given selectively in younger patients with low bleeding risks. It is better if the drug is given hours after the end of the lytic treatment.

REFERENCES

1. The GUSTO Angiographic Investigators. The effects of tissue plasminogen activator, streptokinase, or both on coronary artery patency, ventricular function, and survival after acute myocardial infarction. N Engl J Med 1993; 329: 1615–22

2. Vogt A, von Essen R, Tebbe U, et al. Impact of early perfusion status of the infarct-related artery on short-term mortality after thrombolysis for acute myocardial infarction: retrospective analysis of four German multicenter studies. J Am Coll Cardiol 1993; 21: 1391–5

3. Simes RJ, Topol EJ, Holmes DR, et al. Link between the angiographic substudy and mortality outcomes in a large randomized trial of myocardial perfusion. Importance of early and complete infarct artery reperfusion. GUSTO-I Investigators. Circulation 1995; 91: 1923–8

4. Ross AM, Coyne KS, Moreyra E, et al., for the GUSTO-I Angiographic Investigators. Extended mortality benefit of early postinfarction reperfusion. Circulation 1998; 97: 1549–56

5. Anderson JL, Karagounis LA, Califf RM. Meta-analysis of five reported studies on the relation of early coronary patency grades with mortality and outcomes after acute myocardial infarction. Am J Cardiol 1996; 78: 1–8

6. Califf RM, O'Neill W, Stack RS, et al. Failure of simple clinical measurements to predict perfusion status after intravenous thrombolysis. Ann Intern Med 1988; 108: 658–62

7. Ohman EM, Christenson RH, Califf RM, et al., for the TAMI 7 Study Group. Noninvasive detection of perfusion after thrombolysis based on serum creatine kinase MB changes and clinical variables. Thrombolysis and Angioplasty in Myocardial Infarction. Am Heart J 1993; 126: 819–26

8. Krucoff MW, Croll MA, Pope JE, et al. Continuous 12-lead ST segment recovery analysis in the TAMI 7 study. Performance of a noninvasive method for real-time detection of failed myocardial reperfusion. Circulation 1993; 88: 437–46

9. Shah PK, Cercek B, Lew AS, Ganz W. Angiographic validation of bedside markers of reperfusion. J Am Coll Cardiol 1993; 21: 55–61

10. Sutton AG, Campbell PG, Price DJ, et al. Failure of thrombolysis by streptokinase: detection with a simple electrocardiographic method. Heart 2000; 84: 149–56

11. de Lemos JA, Morrow DA, Gibson CM, et al. TIMI 14 Investigators. Thrombosis In Myocardial Infarction. Early noninvasive detection of failed epicardial reperfusion after fibrinolytic therapy. Am J Cardiol 2001; 88: 353–8

12. Stewart JT, French JK, Theroux P, et al. Early noninvasive identification of failed reperfusion after intravenous thrombolytic therapy in acute myocardial infarction. J Am Coll Cardiol 1998; 31: 1499–1505

13. Tanasijevic MJ, Cannon CP, Antman EM, et al. Myoglobin, creatine-kinase-MB and cardiac troponin-I 60-minute ratios predict infarct-related artery patency after thrombolysis for acute myocardial infarction: results from the Thrombolysis in Myocardial Infarction study (TIMI) 10B. J Am Coll Cardiol 1999; 34: 739–47

14. Morrow DA, Antman EM, Charlesworth A, et al. TIMI risk score for ST elevation myocardial infarction: a convenient, bedside, clinical score for risk assessment at presentation: an intravenous tnPA for treatment of infarcting myocardium early II trial substudy. Circulation 2000; 102: 2031–7

15. Anjaneyulu A, Raghavaraju P, Krishnaswamy R, et al. Demonstration of recanalized left coronary artery after thrombolysis by transthoracic echocardiography. J Am Soc Echocardiogr 2005; 18: 686–92

16. Lee S, Otsuji Y, Minagoe S, et al. Noninvasive evaluation of coronary reperfusion by transthoracic Doppler echocardiography in patients with anterior acute myocardial infarction before coronary intervention. Circulation 2003; 108: 2763–8

17. Kamp O, Lepper W, Vanoverschelde J-L, et al. Serial evaluation of perfusion defects in patients with a first acute myocardial infarction referred for primary PTCA using intravenous myocardial contrast echocardiography. Eur Heart J 2001; 22: 1485–95

18. Wackers FJ, Gibbons RJ, Verani MS, et al. Serial quantitative planar technetium-99m isonitrile imaging in acute myocardial infarction: efficacy for noninvasive assessment of thrombolytic therapy. J Am Coll Cardiol 1989; 14: 861–73

19. Hundley WG, Clarke GD, Landau C, et al. Noninvasive determination of infarct artery patency by cine magnetic resonance angiography. Circulation 1995; 91: 1347–53

20. Meijer A, Verheugt FW, Werter CJ, et al. Aspirin versus coumadin in the prevention of reocclusion and recurrent ischemia after successful thrombolysis: a prospective placebo-controlled angiographic study. Results of the APRICOT Study. Circulation 1993; 87: 1524–30

21. Brouwer MA, Bohncke JR, Veen G, et al. Adverse long-term effects of reocclusion after coronary thrombolysis. J Am Coll Cardiol 1995; 26: 1440–4

22. Single-bolus tenecteplase compared with front-loaded alteplase in acute myocardial infarction: the ASSENT-2 double-blind randomised trial. Assessment of the Safety and Efficacy of a New Thrombolytic Investigators. Lancet 1999; 354: 716–22

23. Gibson CM, Karha J, Murphy SA, et al.; TIMI Study Group. Early and long-term clinical outcomes associated with reinfarction following fibrinolytic administration in the Thrombolysis in Myocardial Infarction trials. J Am Coll Cardiol 2003; 42: 7–16

24. Antman EM, Anbe DT, Armstrong PW, et al. ACC/AHA guidelines for the management of patients with ST elevation myocardial infarction – executive summary: a report of the American College of Cardiology/American Heart Association Task Force on Practice Guidelines (Writing Committee to Revise the 1999 Guidelines for the Management of Patients With Acute Myocardial Infarction). J Am Coll Cardiol 2004; 44: 671–719

25. Langer A, Krucoff MW Klootwijk P, et al., for the GUSTO-I ECG monitoring Substudy Group. Prognostic significance of ST segment shift early after resolution of ST elevation in patients with myocardial infarction treated with thrombolytic therapy: The GUSTO-I ST segment monitoring substudy. J Am Coll Cardiol 1998; 31: 783–9

26. Fung AY, Lai P Topol EJ, et al. Value of percutaneous transluminal coronary angioplasty after unsuccessful intravenous streptokinase therapy in acute myocardial infarction. Am J Cardiol 1986; 58: 686–91

27. Holmes DR Jr, Gersh BJ, Bailey KR, et al. Emergency 'rescue' percutaneous transluminal coronary angioplasty after failed thrombolysis with streptokinase. Early and late results. Circulation 1990; 81: IV51

28. Abbottsmith CW, Topol EJ, George BS, et al. Fate of patients with acute myocardial infarction with patency of the infarct-related vessel achieved with successful thrombolysis versus rescue angioplasty. J Am Coll Cardiol 1990; 16: 770

29. Ellis SG, Van de Werf F, Ribeiro-da Silva E, et al. Present status of rescue coronary angioplasty: current polarization of opinion and randomized trials. J Am Coll Cardiol 1992; 19: 681–6

30. McKendall GR, Forman S, Sopko G, et al. Value of rescue percutaneous transluminal coronary angioplasty following unsuccessful thrombolytic therapy in patients with acute myocardial infarction. Thrombolysis in Myocardial Infarction Investigators. Am J Cardiol 1995; 76: 1108–11

31. Gibson CM, Cannon CP, Greene RM, et al. Rescue angioplasty in the Thrombolysis In Myocardial Infarction (TIMI) 4 trial. Am J Cardiol 1997; 80: 21

32. Schweiger MJ, Cannon CP, Murphy SA, et al. For the TIMI 10B and TIMI 14 Investigators. Early coronary intervention following pharmacologic therapy for acute myocardial infarction (the combined TIMI 10B-TIMI 14 experience). Am J Cardiol 2001; 88: 831–6

33. Belenkie I, Traboulsi M, Hall CA, et al. Rescue angioplasty during myocardial infarction has a beneficial effect on mortality: a tenable hypothesis. Can J Cardiol 1992; 8: 357–62

34. Ellis SG, Ribeiro da Silva E, Heyndrick GR, et al. For the RESCUE Investigators. Randomized comparison of rescue angioplasty with conservative management of patients with early failure of thrombolysis for acute anterior myocardial infarction. Circulation 1994; 90: 2280–4

35. Michels KB, Yusuf S. Does PTCA in acute myocardial infarction affect mortality and reinfarction rates? A quantitative overview (meta-analysis) of the randomized clinical trials. Circulation 1995; 91: 476–85

36. Ellis SG, Lincoff AM, George BS, et al. Randomized evaluation of coronary angioplasty for early TIMI 2 flow after thrombolytic therapy for the treatment of acute myocardial infarction: a new look at an old study. The Thrombolysis and Angioplasty in Myocardial Infarction (TAMI) Study Group. Coron Artery Dis 1994; 5: 611–15

37. Ellis SG, Da Silva ER, Spaulding CM, et al. Review of immediate angioplasty after fibrinolytic therapy for acute myocardial infarction: insights from the RESCUE I, RESCUE II, and other contemporary clinical experiences. Am Heart J 2000; 139: 1046–53

38. Ross AM, Lundergan CF, Rohrbeck SC, et al. Rescue angioplasty after failed thrombolysis: technical and clinical outcomes in a large thrombolysis trial. GUSTO-1 Angiographic Investigators. Global Utilization of Streptokinase and Tissue Plasminogen Activator for Occluded Coronary Arteries. J Am Coll Cardiol 1998; 31: 1511–17

39. Sutton AG, Campbell PG, Graham R, et al. A randomized trial of rescue angioplasty versus a conservative approach for failed fibrinolysis in ST segment elevation myocardial infarction: the Middlesbrough Early Revascularization to Limit INfarction (MERLIN) trial. J Am Coll Cardiol 2004; 44: 287–96

40. Grines CL, O'Neill WW. Rescue angioplasty: does the concept need to be rescued? J Am Coll Cardiol 2004; 44: 297–9

41. Gershlick A. REACT: Rescue Angioplasty versus Conservative Therapy of Repeat Thrombolysis. AHA Scientific Sessions, New Orleans, 2004

42. Topol EJ, Neumann FJ, Montalescot G. A preferred reperfusion strategy for acute myocardial infarction. J Am Coll Cardiol 2003; 42: 1886–7

43. Lefkovits J, Ivanhoe RJ, Califf RM, et al. Effects of platelet glycoprotein IIb/IIIa receptor blockade by a chimeric monoclonal antibody (abciximab) on acute and six-month outcomes after percutaneous coronary angioplasty for acute myocardial infarction. EPIC investigators. Am J Cardiol 1996; 77: 1045–51

44. Sundlof DW, Rerkpattanapitat P, Wongpraparut N, et al. Incidence of bleeding complications associated with abciximab use in conjunction with thrombolytic therapy in patients requiring percutaneous transluminal coronary angioplasty. Am J Cardiol 1999; 83: 1569–71

45. Jong P, Cohen EA, Batchelor W, et al. Bleeding risks with abciximab after full-dose thrombolysis in rescue or urgent angioplasty for acute myocardial infarction. Am Heart J 2001; 141: 218–25

46. Miller JM, Smalling R, Ohman EM, et al. Effectiveness of early coronary angioplasty and abciximab for failed thrombolysis (reteplase or alteplase) during acute myocardial

infarction (results from the GUSTO-III trial). Global Use of Strategies To Open occluded coronary arteries. Am J Cardiol 1999; 84: 779–84

47. The GUSTO V investigators. Reperfusion therapy for acute myocardial infarction with fibrinolytic therapy or combination reduced fibrinolytic therapy and platelet glycoprotein IIb/IIIa inhibition: the GUSTO V randomised trial. Lancet 2001; 357: 1905–14

48. Petronio AS, Musumeci G, Limbruno U, et al. Abciximab improves 6-month clinical outcome after rescue coronary angioplasty. Am Heart J 2002; 143: 334–41

49. Sabatine MS, Cannon CP, Gibson CM, et al., for the CLARITY-TIMI 28 Investigators. Addition of clopidogrel to aspirin and fibrinolytic therapy for myocardial infarction with ST segment elevation. N Engl J Med 2005; 352: 1179–89

50. Mehta SR, Yusuf S, Peters RJG, et al., for the Clopidogrel in Unstable angina to prevent Recurrent Events trial (CURE) Investigators. Effects of pretreatment with clopidogrel and aspirin followed by long-term therapy in patients undergoing percutaneous coronary intervention: the PCI-CURE study. Lancet 2001; 358: 527–33

51. Steinhubl SR, Berger PB, Mann JT, et al. Early and sustained dual oral antiplatelet therapy following percutaneous coronary intervention: a randomized controlled trial. J Am Med Assoc 2002; 288: 2411–20

52. Garot P, Himbert D, Juliard JM, et al. Incidence, consequences, and risk factors of early reocclusion after primary and/or rescue percutaneous transluminal coronary angioplasty for acute myocardial infarction. Am J Cardiol 1998; 82: 554–8

53. Moreno R, Garcia E, Abeytua M, et al. Coronary stenting during rescue angioplasty after failed thrombolysis. Catheter Cardiovasc Interv 1999; 47: 1–5

54. Cafri C, Denktas AE, Crystal E, Ilia R, Battler A. Contribution of stenting to the results of rescue PTCA. Catheter Cardiovasc Interv 1999; 47: 411–14

55. Dauerman HL, Prpic R, Andreou C, Vu MA, Popma JJ. Angiographic and clinical outcomes after rescue coronary stenting. Catheter Cardiovasc Interv 2000; 50: 269–75

56. Schomig A, Ndrepepa G, Mehilli J, et al.; STOPAMI-4 study investigators. A randomized trial of coronary stenting versus balloon angioplasty as a rescue intervention after failed thrombolysis in patients with acute myocardial infarction. J Am Coll Cardiol 2004; 44: 2073–9

57. Ohman EM, George BS, White CJ, et al. Use of aortic counterpulsation to improve sustained coronary artery patency during acute myocardial infarction. Results of a randomized trial. The Randomized IABP Study Group. Circulation 1994; 90: 792–9

58. Ishihara M, Sato H, Tateishi H, et al. Intraaortic balloon pumping as an adjunctive therapy to rescue coronary angioplasty after failed thrombolysis in anterior wall myocardial infarction. Am J Cardiol 1995; 76: 73–5

59. Richardson SG, Allen DC, Morton P, Murtagh JG, Scott ME, O'Keeffe DB. Pathological changes after intravenous streptokinase treatment in eight patients with acute myocardial infarction. Br Heart J 1989; 61: 390–5

60. Lee CH, Tan HC, Teo SG, Sutandar A, Lim YT. Safety and feasibility of X-sizer-facilitated rescue percutaneous coronary intervention: a preliminary experience. J Invasive Cardiol 2005; 17: 1–4

61. Yip HK, Wu CJ, Chang HW, et al. Effect of the PercuSurge GuardWire device on the integrity of microvasculature and clinical outcomes during primary transradial coronary intervention in acute myocardial infarction. Am J Cardiol 2003; 92: 1331–5

62. Orrego PS, Delgado A, Piccalo G, Salvade P, Bonacina E, Klugmann S. Distal protection in native coronary arteries during primary angioplasty in acute myocardial infarction: single-center experience. Catheter Cardiovasc Interv 2003; 60: 152–8

63. Huang Z, Katoh O, Nakamura S, Negoro S, Kobayashi T, Tanigawa J. Evaluation of the PercuSurge Guardwire Plus Temporary Occlusion and Aspiration System during primary angioplasty in acute myocardial infarction. Catheter Cardiovasc Interv 2003; 60: 443–51

64. Stone GW, Webb J, Cox DA, et al.; Enhanced Myocardial Efficacy and Recovery by Aspiration of Liberated Debris (EMERALD) Investigators. Distal microcirculatory protection during percutaneous coronary intervention in acute ST segment elevation myocardial infarction: a randomized controlled trial. J Am Med Assoc 2005; 293: 1063–72

65. Kassam S, Cantor WJ, Patel D, et al. Radial versus femoral access for rescue percutaneous coronary intervention with adjuvant glycoprotein IIb/IIIa inhibitor use. Can J Cardiol 2004; 20: 1439–42

Index

Page numbers in italic refer to figures or tables.